W9-AOU-000

Epilepsy and the Family

Epilepsy and the Family

Richard Lechtenberg, M.D.

Harvard University Press

Cambridge, Massachusetts, and London, England

Library of Congress Cataloging in Publication Data
Lechtenberg, Richard.
  Epilepsy and the family.
  Includes bibliographical references and index.
  1. Epileptics—Family relationships. 2. Epilepsy—
Psychological aspects. 3. Epilepsy—Social aspects.
I. Title.
RC372.L38   1984   362.1'96853   84-6714
ISBN 0-674-25888-6 (alk. paper) (cloth)
ISBN 0-674-25889-4 (paper)

To Dr. Sydney S. Gellis

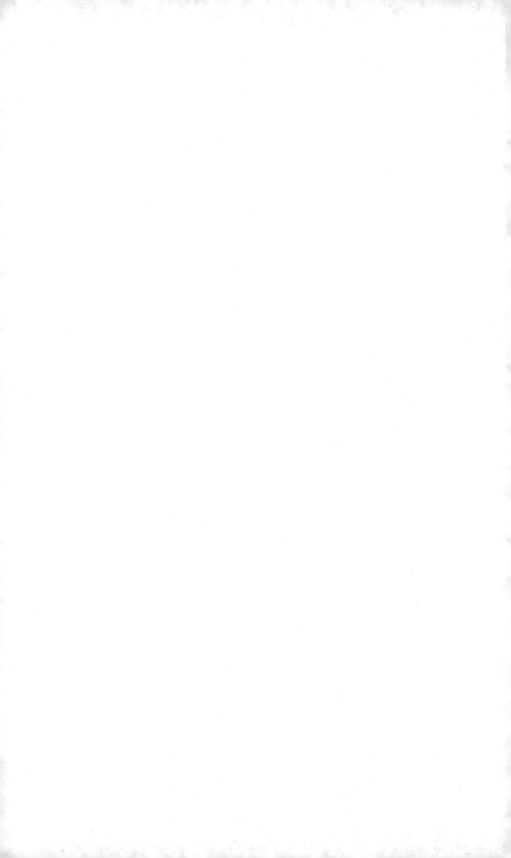

Acknowledgments

I want to thank Lois Akner, M.S.W., for her contributions as a family therapist to this study. Albert R. Paglialunga provided photographs from which Shelly E. Eshleman drew the sketches for this book. Luisa Karoly supplied electroencephalograms, and Dr. Roger Cracco provided advice on and interpretation of the electroencephalograms. Susan Wallace gave me invaluable editorial comments and recommendations. The most important contributors to this book were the many families who brought me their problems and questions and asked for answers.

Contents

Epilepsy and the Family

Chapter 1

Epilepsy: Its Characteristics and Impact

Patrick was interested in a career in medicine because his father had epilepsy. Although the seizures frightened him at first, he quickly learned how to help his father when an attack occurred. He also advised friends and relatives what to do and what not to do during these attacks. If young children were present, he would reassure them that the seizure was frightening but not dangerous. His father admitted that he relied heavily upon his son, and that without Patrick's keen sense of when a seizure was about to occur he would have suffered many more injuries than he did. Patrick was 3 years old at the time.

Miriam's young son, David, had had seizures since birth and had undergone several operations to treat birth defects associated with the epilepsy. Even with his mother's constant attention, David had as many as fifteen seizures a day. Miriam was obsessed with the dangers he faced every time he had a seizure. Her husband understood her preoccupation with David and spent all his spare time helping with his supervision and medications. Even so, the child took up all of Miriam's time and attention. Their four other children had to look after themselves.

Elizabeth married a man who had his first seizure a few days before their wedding. The epilepsy soon became intractable despite a variety of medications and other less conventional treatments. Elizabeth's every action had to take her husband's disorder into account. Her thorough preoccupation with it became clear when she went to renew her driver's license. Looking at the form she had filled out, the clerk asked her to answer additional questions about her epilepsy. After a moment of confusion she realized that she had indicated on the form that she was impaired by epilepsy. Even after the error was pointed out, Elizabeth felt that her answer was quite accurate: her husband's epilepsy was as much an impairment for her as for him.

Epilepsy, like any chronic medical problem, affects not only the person suffering from it but that person's family as well. Parents whose child develops epilepsy must cope with special restrictions, constant medication, and perhaps learning or behavior problems. Other children in the family may be deprived of their parents' attention because of the extra needs of the epileptic child. A wife may find that after her husband develops epilepsy he can no longer support the family or loses interest in sex.

The impact of epilepsy on a particular family partly depends on the type and frequency of the seizures. But even well-controlled epilepsy, in which the victim hardly ever has seizures, can be quite disruptive. Even if the person with epilepsy has been free of seizures for months or years, the family may not be able to forget the threat of renewed seizures. The fact that a family member has a seizure disorder often remains a major consideration in the family's plans and activities. Parents may obsessively shelter their epileptic child. The husband of a woman who has only occasional seizures may harbor doubts that his wife can be relied upon in a crisis. The entire family may treat the person with epilepsy as "sick" even after decades without seizures.

If the epilepsy is poorly controlled, so that the victim has frequent and unpredictable seizures, it can destabilize the family and drain its financial and emotional resources. What circumstances are thought to bring on seizures may take on almost magical significance, and the family will go to great lengths to avoid them. If social life seems to bring on a young girl's seizures, her parents may forbid her to see her friends. A couple may decide not to have a second child because the wife had more frequent seizures during her first pregnancy. Many families fear that any change in lifestyle, however slight, may touch off a new round of seizures. As a result, family interactions can become desperately rigid. The person with epilepsy is often surrounded by tensions even if all members of the family insist that the epilepsy is not a significant problem.

The goal for every person with epilepsy is to lead as normal a life as possible. Ideally, this is a life without seizures; if this cannot be achieved it is at least a life free of unreasonable fears or prohibitions. The family helps to determine what kind of life the epileptic person will live. Lowered expectations can become self-fulfilling prophecies. An adult who is expected to take little responsibility within the family because of having epilepsy often lives up to that expectation. An overprotected child will grow up to be an unprepared adult. A person who has always been treated as "sick" will have trouble realizing his or her own capabilities. Most people with epilepsy are able to lead virtually normal lives. Informed and understanding families are vitally important in helping them to do so.

Characteristics of Epilepsy

Epilepsy occurs in men, women, and children of every culture. In the United States it affects at least one out of every two hundred people. It is a disturbance of the nervous system that abruptly interferes with behavior, perception, movement, consciousness, or other brain functions. Individual attacks are called seizures; when the attacks occur repeatedly, the problem is called a seizure disorder or epilepsy. Because of the stigma attached to the term *epilepsy*, some physicians avoid using it. Patients may be told instead that they have seizures, fits, or a seizure disorder—all synonyms for epilepsy. The term "convulsion" is usually reserved for seizures in which jerking of the limbs or trunk and loss of consciousness are prominent features. Seizures are so commonly referred to as convulsions that physicians routinely call medications to suppress seizure activity anticonvulsants. Anticonvulsants are antiepileptic medications used for all types of seizures.

Inappropriate electrical activity in the brain is the basis for all seizure disorders, though the different types of epilepsy often have little more in common than this. Nerve cells in the brain communicate and regulate each other's activity primarily by way of electrical signals running along fine extensions from the body of one nerve cell, or neuron, that make contact with the bodies of or projections from other nerve cells (Figure 1.1). Seizures occur when there is a disorganized or untimely discharge of electrical impulses from many nerve cells, particularly in the superficial layers of the brain called the cerebral cortex. Coordinated or at least somewhat disciplined activity of nerve cells in this part of the brain is essential for normal consciousness, sensation, strength, and coordination. During a seizure, one or all of these brain functions may be affected to varying degrees. In some types of epilepsy seizures cause loss of consciousness,

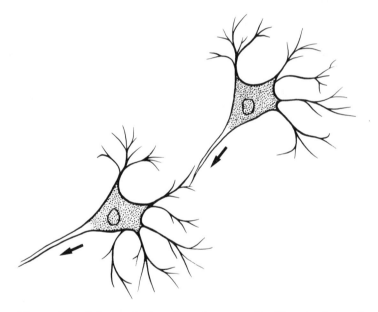

Figure 1.1 Schematic drawing of nerve cells. Electrical signals travel along projections to and from nerve cells (arrows) to transmit information from one part of the brain to another. The brain has millions of cells forming complex circuits. The message traveling from one cell to another may either inhibit or excite the nerve cell receiving the signal.

whereas in others consciousness is impaired minimally, if at all. Some types of seizures invariably include visual or auditory hallucinations, and others never produce changes in vision, hearing, smell, taste, or other sensations. Although there are many different types of epilepsy, most people with a seizure disorder experience only one type of seizure.

Misconceptions and misunderstandings develop because epilepsy is not a single entity with simple characteristics. A businessman who developed seizures after a head injury insisted for several years that he did not have epilepsy because his episodes of altered consciousness involved wandering, peculiar movements and behavior, and temporary loss of memory, but no jerking of his arms and legs. He insisted that a person with epilepsy always fell down, lost consciousness, and jerked his arms and legs. What he recognized as epilepsy—and what many laymen consider to be epilepsy—is generalized tonic-clonic, or so-called grand mal, epilepsy. The type of seizure disorder that he had was complex partial, or so-called psychomotor, epilepsy. This common misconception about epilepsy allowed the businessman to deny having a condition he feared; he preferred to believe he had an emotional disorder. Though there was little in his particular seizure episodes to suggest a psychological problem, some types of epilepsy are indeed difficult to distinguish from psychiatric disease without rigorous neurologic testing.

This businessman's denial that he had epilepsy is a common response, but there is no way you anticipate how an individual will react to the diagnosis of epilepsy. A 25-year-old medical technician with transient episodes of numbness on one side of her body was relieved to discover that her problem was an unusual type of seizure disorder called focal sensory epilepsy. She had feared that the peculiar sensations were evidence of mental illness, and unlike the businessman she found the prospect of a psychiatric problem much more terrifying than a neurologic problem.

Although there are many types of seizure disorders, some characteristics appear with striking frequency, and some attacks are virtually identical for many people. Because stereotyped features do recur in different individuals, seizures can be classified into broad categories (see Box 1.1). Some types of seizures, such as the so-called petit mal (generalized nonconvulsive) episodes of childhood, tend to be remarkably consistent from person to person and therefore easily recognized, whereas other seizures, such as the psychomotor (complex partial) episodes that occur at any age, are extremely diverse and therefore more difficult to identify with confidence. Deciding what specific form of epilepsy an individual suffers from may not be simple, but making an accurate diagnosis is important for proper treatment and for anticipating problems.

Provocative Stimuli and Seizure Thresholds

Epilepsy by definition involves *recurrent* seizure activity or at least recurrent *risk* of seizure activity. The first seizure an individual has does not necessarily mean the individual has epilepsy. An isolated seizure may be nothing more than a passing response to a head injury, a nervous system infection, or a metabolic imbalance; after recovering from these conditions, the person may never be at risk for another seizure. For example, pregnant women occasionally develop a disorder called toxemia, which in its most serious form can lead to one or several seizures. One would not say, however, that these women suffer from epilepsy, since they are not at risk under normal circumstances, namely when they are not pregnant and are not also suffering from toxemia. In fact, anyone, however normal his or her nervous system, can be induced to have a seizure if subjected to

---

Box 1.1
Types of Epilepsy

Generalized: Convulsive and nonconvulsive

Partial: Elementary and complex

adequately provocative stimuli, such as an electrical shock to the brain.[1]

Epilepsy itself is not a hereditary problem, but there are nervous system disorders that can be inherited and can cause seizures. In some individuals one seizure may be evidence of a hereditary problem that will cause intractable epilepsy in other members of the family. With antiepileptic medication, the person who has had only one seizure may remain seizure-free forever. That person nevertheless has epilepsy, because the risk, as evidenced in other members of the family, of recurrent seizures is still present. Some people will have only one seizure even without medication, even if they have a hereditary disease that often causes seizures. These people are spared further attacks either because they are not as vulnerable to stimuli that evoke seizures as are other people in their families or because they are almost never exposed to the stimuli to which they are vulnerable.

What will trigger seizures in people with epilepsy is as variable as the form the seizure activity may assume. Starvation, dehydration, and exhaustion may be required to provoke attacks in one person, while a single night without much sleep may provoke seizures in another person with the same type of epilepsy. In most cases there is no obvious explanation for the difference. Even closely related people whose hereditary problem makes them seizure-prone may require dramatically different conditions for seizures to occur. One child with generalized tonic-clonic (grand mal) convulsions that develop only after several days of sleep deprivation may have a brother whose seizures occur whenever he sees a flashing light.

Sleeplessness, physical exhaustion, trauma, infection, and alcohol abuse are common precipitants of recurrent seizures in individuals with well-controlled epilepsy (see Box 1.2). But the most frequent causes of recurrent seizures is erratic use of antiepileptic drugs. All of these provocative situations and stimuli must be avoided to minimize the risk of seizures. For most people this simply means developing daily routines that eliminate irregular hours and excessive burdens. It is also important to pay extra attention to personal health and hygiene; otherwise, dental

---

Box 1.2
Provocative Stimuli

Anticonvulsant noncompliance

Sleep deprivation

Trauma

Alcohol withdrawal

Barbiturate withdrawal

Amphetamine abuse

Flashing lights

---

problems, foot infections, viral syndromes, and other common illnesses can lead to seizures. For example, nocturnal seizures may be the first indication of a smoldering gum infection. Well-concealed alcohol abuse occasionally explains uncontrollable seizure activity that disappears when the alcoholic is admitted to a hospital for closer observation. Abuse of other drugs, such as amphetamines and barbiturates, may also trigger seizures.

Many women with epilepsy notice an increase in seizures at about the time of menstruation. The hormonal changes of the menstrual cycle are not easily avoided. But adjusting a woman's dose of anticonvulsant medication in anticipation of a monthly peak in susceptibility to seizures may keep her free of seizures. These adjustments to the menstrual cycle become unnecessary after menopause.

Less common, but more disturbing, are so-called reflex epilepsies, in which seizures may be triggered by nothing more than a specific noise, sight, action, or even thought. As routine and unavoidable an activity as eating initiates seizures in some people. One young man with post-traumatic complex partial (psychomotor) seizures would develop a generalized convulsion whenever he looked to the left if he did not turn his head while shifting his eyes. In time, most individuals learn what will trigger their seizures and try to avoid those provocative stimuli.[2]

A person who is vulnerable to seizures is said to have a lowered *seizure threshold*. As already mentioned, the threshold may be only temporarily lowered, so that just one seizure occurs in a lifetime; or it may be chronically lowered, so that the person is vulnerable to seizures under conditions that normal people can tolerate uneventfully. Certain structural and metabolic abnormalities in the brain will predictably lower seizure thresholds. A brain tumor, a vascular malformation, or a central nervous system infection will invariably increase an individual's susceptibility to seizure activity. A seizure disorder may also develop after head injury in an automobile accident or after brain damage from a stroke. Epilepsy may be the first sign of the problem, or seizures may fail to develop even when the damage to the nervous system is substantial. For example, the infant son of a man with tuberous sclerosis—a hereditary disease causing changes in the brain, skin, and other organs—had severe mental retardation and uncontrollable seizures, whereas his father, who had less dramatic manifestations of the disease, was a successful mathematician and university professor. When the cause of the lowered seizure threshold produces other signs of impaired functioning of the nervous system, such as mental retardation, these other symptoms help to explain why the individual has a seizure disorder.

If epilepsy is only one symptom of an underlying problem—which may be a head injury, meningitis, stroke, a metabolic problem, or tumor—the epilepsy is called *symptomatic*. Where there is no apparent damage or disease responsible for the seizures—no obvious brain damage and no associated neurologic signs—the disorder is called *idiopathic epilepsy*, meaning that we simply do not know what causes it. People with idiopathic epilepsy are assumed to have subtle abnormalities in the structure or metabolism of the brain that are beyond the resolution of techniques currently available for investigating these aspects of the nervous system. Symptomatic and idiopathic epilepsies differ in several respects, including their natural histories and responses to treatment.

Epilepsy as a Chronic Disease

Many of the social and psychological problems that develop around epilepsy also occur with other chronic health problems, but epilepsy poses special problems for both the individuals affected and people intimately involved with them. Much of epilepsy's disruptive force comes from its unpredictability. Epilepsy is more often a *threat* than an active condition. Unlike chronic heart, liver, kidney, or lung disease, it does not follow relatively consistent patterns that can be used to make long-term, as well as short-term, decisions about schooling, work, marriage, and reproduction. Even at its worst, epilepsy is rarely lethal and usually does not cause progressive disability; rather, the disability associated with epilepsy is transient and unpredictable.

The need to take one or several medications every day is as much a nuisance with epilepsy as it is in any chronic illness, but the advantages provided by the drugs are much less obvious in the patient with seizures than in the patient with congestive heart failure or chronic kidney disease. A person with chest pain and inability to exercise caused by a cardiac problem can easily recognize the benefits of taking the prescribed medications. With epilepsy, control of the seizures is never certain, even on an ideal dose of anticonvulsant medication, and the side effects of these antiepileptic drugs can be all too obvious.

Although perfect control of seizures is elusive, they can be well controlled with medication in more than 80 percent of patients with epilepsy. Unfortunately, many people with infrequent seizures are unwilling to be chained to medication for years or decades. Even when their seizures are not well controlled, some patients may simply give up on the medication, in an irrational attempt to shed the sick role that permeates their lives. However, rejecting treatment only compromises their lives further when seizures reappear. The family's belief that the affected member requires special consideration and lowered expectations is reinforced by this apparently self-destructive behavior.

People with epilepsy are often compelled to explain behavior they exhibit involuntarily (Box 1.3). With complex partial (psychomotor) epilepsy, some individuals make peculiar noises, defecate, or obsessively drink water during the period of altered consciousness. When they regain normal consciousness they do not understand why they acted in these socially inappropriate ways, but the people around them may be unwilling to believe the behavior was not intentional. Even when the seizure disorder is recognized, the burden on the person suffering from the seizures remain. An unsympathetic family may demand justification of inappropriate behavior long after the behavior is ascribed to a neurologic problem.

Common Misconceptions

Complicating the treatment of any individual with epilepsy are the popular misconceptions that surround this particular chronic disease. Less than forty years ago a British medical journal indicated that the general public believed people with epilepsy were "mentally imbalanced, dull, or frankly mentally defective, liable to progressive mental deterioration, awkward to live with, antisocial or potentially criminal, incurable, . . . unemployable, and persons who should be sequestered in institutions." These

---

Box 1.3
Common Initial Signs of Epilepsy

Staring spells

Bedwetting

Memory gaps

Wandering

Nocturnal tongue-biting

Violent muscle spasms in sleep

notions are much less pervasive today than they were thirty or forty years ago. Nonetheless, epilepsy still is often viewed as a type of insanity, and it is routinely presumed to be hereditary.[3]

Many family members and employers worry that violent behavior will occur with epileptic attacks. This misconception has been fostered by the dramatic mood shifts that do occur in some seizure disorders and by a few highly publicized court cases claiming epilepsy as a basis for antisocial or criminal behavior. Another common notion is that brain damage and epilepsy are inextricably linked. Even if the affected individual has no intellectual impairment, significant brain damage is often presumed to be an unavoidable concomitant of the epilepsy. This view probably survives because people with severe brain damage often do develop seizures as one of the signs of the damage. However, this does not mean that everyone with epilepsy is intellectually impaired. With idiopathic epilepsy, in fact, intellectual impairment is unusual.

Although individuals with seizures soon recognize that these common notions of epilepsy are inaccurate, they also realize that it is to their advantage to conceal their disorder. Attempting to convince friends and employers that the seizures do not indicate a mental or emotional defect often exposes the epileptic individual to further penalties for frankness.

The Struggle to Conceal Epilepsy

Simply labeling an individual as epileptic often causes considerable social damage. Once recognized as having epilepsy, the individual loses his or her driver's license. Life insurance becomes difficult to secure, and health insurance is expensive. Forty percent of individuals with epilepsy have problems finding jobs and almost 20 percent of parents whose children do not suffer from epilepsy are opposed to the idea of their children marrying individuals with epilepsy. It is no wonder that many people with epilepsy go to great lengths to conceal their disorder.[4]

Patients with low seizure thresholds may risk recurrent seizures by not taking their medication at the prescribed times of day if taking the medication would arouse questions. A young woman with generalized convulsions was advised not to drink alcohol because of possible interactions with her anticonvulsants. After four years of good drug compliance, she abruptly stopped taking the medication because her friends asked why she did not drink alcohol. Rather than increase suspicions about her health, she heeded her physician's advice to avoid mixing alcohol and anticonvulsants by eliminating the anticonvulsants. To avoid being reprimanded by her physician for risking a recurrence of seizures she stopped going to doctors.

Many young adults conceal their epilepsy out of concern about rejection by potential spouses. As marriage becomes likely, revealing the neurologic problem becomes even more difficult. If a seizure occurs during the engagement or shortly after the marriage, the uninformed partner may abandon the person with epilepsy, often because of the shock and deception as much as the seizure disorder itself.

The most common setting for concealment of epilepsy is in the workplace. Curiously, people involved in manual labor are more likely to notify employers of their neurologic problem than individuals working in managerial or other white-collar positions. An executive with epilepsy faces more resistance to advancement than a carpenter with the same disease, even though the manual laborer runs a greater risk of mishap because of his epilepsy than does the executive. Presumably, the common misconception that thinking cannot be completely normal in someone who has epilepsy interferes with the executive's advancement, whereas skill at manual tasks is routinely perceived as less dependent upon intellectual discipline.[5]

Types of Epilepsy

Accurately identifying the type of epilepsy an individual has is the first step in treating the disorder. If an underlying condition, such as a nervous system infection or a tumor, is responsible for the seizures, it must be eliminated or managed as part of the treatment. Even if no basis for the epilepsy can be found, the seizures can usually be treated and controlled if the drugs used are appropriate for the type of epilepsy the patient has. In fact, the majority of seizure disorders remain unexplained even after extensive investigation. As with any diagnosis, the conclusion that the seizures are not symptomatic of an injury to the brain or a metabolic problem is nothing more than the best guess that can be made based on the information available. The cause of an "idiopathic" epilepsy may become apparent long after the initial evaluation. A slowly growing tumor may produce nothing more than seizures for years; a metabolic disease involving the brain may cause seizures initially and intellectual impairment years later. Fortunately, these insidious problems are rarely the explanation for an idiopathic seizure disorder. Most seizure disorders that cannot be explained after routine neurologic tests remain unexplained for the rest of the person's life.

Identifying the type of seizure provides valuable information to the physician, patient, and family. Children with generalized absence (petit mal) epilepsy have problems and prognoses (predicted outcomes) very different from those of children with complex partial (psychomotor) epilepsy, even though both groups of children may have little more than staring spells as evidence of the epilepsy. The treatment and inconvenience of complex partial seizures in adults are distinct from those of generalized tonic-clonic (grand mal) seizures, even though both are routinely associated with profoundly altered consciousness.

Several features of a person's seizure disorder determine what type of epilepsy the person has. The patient's age, the area of the brain that is most disturbed by abnormal electrical activity, the sequence of physical and mental changes that occur during the seizure, and the form of electroencephalographic (brain wave) recordings during the seizure all enter into the classification of the seizure type. In many cases, a full and accurate description of the symptoms and signs before, during, and after the epileptic attack provides enough information for the physician to identify the seizure disorder. Unfortunately, the reports of patients experiencing the attacks and of families or friends witnessing them are usually incomplete or inaccurate. The individual with epilepsy is confused, and relatives and friends are invariably frightened or upset. Brain wave changes associated with a seizure are much more objective, but obtaining a recording before, during, and after an episode is difficult, if not impossible, with patients who have infrequent seizures. Because of this, the physician's initial impression of the type of epilepsy affecting the patient may be revised as more information about the episodes becomes available.

Generalized Seizures

Most seizure disorders can be defined as either generalized or partial (see Box 1.4). With generalized seizures, both sides of the brain seem to be disturbed simultaneously by abnormal electrical activity. In partial seizures, a local abnormality spreads to involve both sides of the brain or stays limited to part of the cerebrum (see Figure 1.2). The patient with a generalized seizure will lose consciousness for seconds or hours, a lapse sometimes more obvious to others than to the affected person. The most common types of generalized seizures are the tonic-clonic (or grand mal) and absence (or petit mal) forms.[6]

GENERALIZED TONIC-CLONIC EPILEPSY *(Convulsive, Grand Mal Seizures)*. Generalized convulsive (grand mal) seizures can develop at any age. The affected person has an abrupt loss of consciousness followed by convulsive movements of the body. These convulsive movements are called tonic-clonic because there are two phases of muscle activity, one in which limb and trunk muscles become extremely rigid as they persistently, or tonically, enter a violent spasm of activity, and one in which the muscles contract rhythmically, that is, clonically. In the tonic phase the patient may arch his back or forcefully keep his arms and legs parallel to his trunk. Changes in breathing may be obvious and may produce gasping noises and a bluish complexion. These changes give the false impression that the seizure victim is suffocating. Such worrisome signs routinely pass in a matter of seconds, and a patient's color returns to normal. In the clonic phase the limbs and trunk jerk or thrash about as muscle contractions become rhythmical and intermittent. This type of seizure activity is usually called a convulsion (Box 1.5).

**Box 1.4
Seizure Types**

Proper Name	*Common Name*
Generalized	
Tonic-clonic or convulsive	Grand mal Major motor
Clonic	
Tonic	
Absence or nonconvulsive*	Petit mal Absence
Infantile spasms*	
Atonic and akinetic*	Drop attacks
Myoclonic*	
Partial	
Simple or elementary	
Motor	Focal motor Jacksonian
Sensory	Focal sensory Special sensory
Complex with or without impaired consciousness	Psychomotor Temporal lobe
Secondarily generalized	

*Also called minor motor seizures.

Tongue biting and urination often occur during grand mal seizures. Even when the tongue is not bitten, the gums or cheek may suffer minor cuts from involuntary jaw movements. The

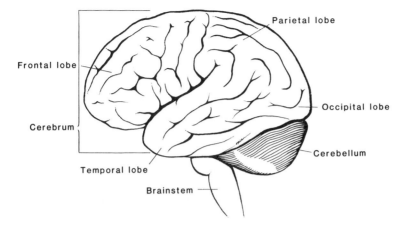

Figure 1.2 Principal divisions of the brain. The cerebrum is the part of the brain most disturbed when a seizure occurs. The most superficial layers of nerve cells in the cerebrum are called the cortex. The cerebellum is primarily responsible for the coordination of movements. Information from the brain travels to different parts of the body through the brainstem and the spinal cord. The spinal cord is an extention of the brainstem. All of the structures indicated on this diagram are inside the skull.

patient may also defecate or forcefully kick nearby objects. Violent contractions of the muscles about the shoulder may dislocate the arm at the shoulder joint. Elderly individuals occasionally develop spine fractures from the force of spinal muscle contractions, but most people with this type of seizure do not hurt themselves unless they suffer an injury during the initial collapse to the ground.

These attacks routinely appear with little or no warning. If there is a warning, it is usually little more than a few seconds of malaise or lightheadedness preceding the episode. The acute epileptic (ictal) phenomena last several seconds to a few minutes. Subsequently, the patient will be poorly responsive to all stimuli for minutes or hours. This interval of impaired consciousness is called the postictal period. If this type of seizure occurs while the person with epilepsy is sleeping, he may wonder why his tongue is sore or why there is urine in his bed, but not

---

Box 1.5
Features of generalized tonic-clonic
(grand mal) seizures

Little or no warning of impending seizure

Electroencephalogram diffusely abnormal at start

Loss of posture with high risk of self-injury

Loss of consciousness

Bladder or bowel incontinence likely

Violent contraction of limb and trunk muscles

Postictal confusion lasting minutes

---

realize that he had a seizure. Children who develop seizures during sleep may be punished for bedwetting or referred for psychiatric evaluation before a seizure disorder is recognized. An adult's bed partner may be kicked during the clonic phase of the seizure and stop sleeping in the same bed with the epileptic person because of what is interpreted as restlessness.

Most people do not grow out of this type of epilepsy. That is, simply growing older does not improve one's chances of remission, nor does the character of the seizure usually change with age. Seizure activity may be inapparent for years and then recur for no obvious reason. But, as discussed in Chapter 11, antiepileptic drugs are usually effective in suppressing the convulsions in most people with this type of epilepsy.

GENERALIZED ABSENCE EPILEPSY *(Petit Mal Seizures or Absence Attacks)*. The patient with generalized absence epilepsy is usually a child, and the principal feature of the seizure disorder is a momentary loss of consciousness (Box 1.6). Seizures usually appear at 6 to 12 years of age and disappear or change to another type by the end of adolescence. The seizures may not

---

Box 1.6
Features of generalized absence
(petit mal) seizures

No warning of impending seizure

Electroencephalogram with typical 3-per-second
spike-and-slow-wave pattern

No loss of posture

Loss of consciousness

No bladder or bowel incontinence

No violent limb or trunk movements

No postictal confusion

---

be recognized for years because the child's absence attacks may not be thought to be anything more than peculiar behavior. The child abruptly becomes inattentive and may stop talking in the middle of a sentence without even realizing the interruption in speech has occurred. During the seizures, these children do not fall down, jerk their limbs, or thrash about. They may blink or make other subtle facial movements, but more characteristic is an interruption of any movements that were occurring. A child who is sitting or standing when the attack occurs remains sitting or standing. The brain wave pattern in children with this type of epilepsy is very helpful in establishing the diagnosis (Figure 1.3).[7]

Transient loss of consciousness, the principal manifestation of petit mal epilepsy, is also a common feature of psychomotor (complex partial) epilepsy. When petit mal epilepsy is responsible for the absence attacks, the return to normal consciousness is just as abrupt as the loss of consciousness. There is usually no confusion or lethargy following the seizure. The child may not even realize that he or she has had an episode of altered

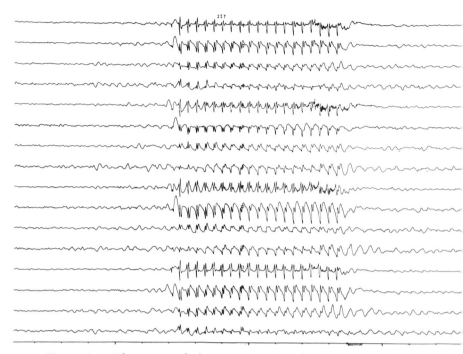

Figure 1.3 Electroencephalogram in petit mal epilepsy. The 3-per-second spike-and-slow-wave discharges that are characteristic of generalized absence (petit mal) epilepsy occupy the middle third of this 17-second recording. The child had a staring spell and was mute when these brain waves appeared.

consciousness. When psychomotor seizures are responsible, in contrast, the child does not abruptly return to normal consciousness but goes through a period of inattentiveness or confusion that may last minutes or hours.

Although petit mal seizures that start in childhood sometimes persist through adolescence and into adult life, they usually evolve into more complex seizures. The petit mal seizures are replaced by psychomotor or grand mal epilepsy as the child becomes an adult. Occasionally the absence attacks persist in association with other types of seizures. Adults with no history of childhood seizures who develop absence attacks (epileptic staring spells) do not have petit mal epilepsy, but may have another type of seizure disorder, such as psychomotor (complex partial) epilepsy.

OTHER GENERALIZED SEIZURES. There are several other types of generalized seizures, but they are much less common than grand mal and petit mal seizures. Infants with profoundly abnormal electroencephalograms and frequent convulsive spasms that jerk their entire bodies are said to have infantile spasms. The profoundly abnormal pattern of brain waves that persists even between apparent spasms, called *hypsarrhythmia*, is a sign of diffusely abnormal brain activity. Infantile spasms with hypsarrhythmia are caused by several different types of injury to the brain, but they most often develop if the child suffers trauma or inadequate oxygen (asphyxia) at birth. This type of generalized seizure disorder invariably develops between birth and 3 years of age and is usually associated with mental retardation or other obvious signs of irreversible brain damage.[8]

Less common forms of generalized seizures include transient attacks of massive muscle jerks (myoclonic seizures) that may literally throw the affected individual to the ground, and fleeting episodes of impaired body tone (atonic attacks) that are generally seen only in infants. In each of these generalized seizure disorders a metabolic or structural problem in the central nervous system must be carefully sought before the seizures are considered idiopathic.

Partial Seizures

With partial seizures, abnormal electrical activity always starts in a limited and usually discernible area of the cerebral cortex. During the seizure, the abnormal activity spreads and may even generalize to involve much of the cerebral cortex. When this happens within a few seconds, the seizure resembles a generalized seizure. The only way to identify these seizures as partial—or, more accurately, sequential—seizures is by following the spread of abnormal electrical activity on an electroencephalographic recording obtained during the seizure.[9]

Partial epilepsies assume two basic forms, elementary (or simple) and complex. When the seizure activity causes abnormal sensation or movement that is limited to one part of the body or disturbed perceptions involving only one sense, it is classified as a partial seizure with elementary or simple symptomatology (see Box 1.4). This is better known as focal motor or focal sensory epilepsy. Partial seizures that cause changes in behavior, sensation, and movement in a variety of combinations are generally known as psychomotor or complex partial seizures.

COMPLEX PARTIAL *(Psychomotor, Temporal Lobe)* EPILEPSY. Complex partial epilepsy is the most common of the partial epilepsies. Twenty to thirty percent of all people suffering from seizures have this type. The first attack usually occurs at about the time of puberty, but prepubertal children and adults of all ages can also develop complex partial seizures. One-third of patients with psychomotor seizures develop typical attacks only after years of generalized epilepsy (grand mal or petit mal). Sixty-four percent of people with complex partial seizures have generalized seizures as well.[10]

Most complex partial seizures begin in the temporal lobe of the brain, and significant structural damage in the temporal lobe can be found in some patients. But for most, there is no obvious structural problem responsible for the psychomotor seizures. Even in these cases, though, the focus of epileptic activity defined by electroencephalographic studies is usually in the temporal lobe, and therefore, these seizures are also called temporal lobe seizures. This is a misleading name, in that abnormal electrical activity arising in the temporal lobe can produce other kinds of seizures besides psychomotor, and some psychomotor seizures begin outside the temporal lobe. Nevertheless, temporal lobe epilepsy is a very old term, and, like grand mal and petit mal, it is still widely used.[11]

Complex partial seizures are often difficult to recognize because of the variety of abnormal behaviors shown by people with this disorder (Box 1.7). This variability often leads friends, family members, and even physicians caring for the patient to suspect a psychological basis for much, if not all, of the abnormal behavior observed. Some patients with psychomotor epilepsy

---

Box 1.7
Features of complex partial seizures
(psychomotor or temporal lobe)

Often has aura warning of impending seizure

Electroencephalogram shows abnormality
starting locally

May have loss of posture or abnormal
limb movments

May have altered or complete loss
of consciousness

May have prominent emotional or thought
disorder during seizure

Postictal confusion likely to persist
minutes to hours

---

do have psychiatric problems distinct from their seizure disorders, but most do not.

Every seizure, whether generalized or partial, has several discrete stages, but the stages are especially obvious with complex partial seizures. The stage with the most dramatic electrical disorganization is called the *ictus* of the seizure. This is often preceded by some type of warning, called the *aura*. The aura is actually part of the seizure proper, even though most patients perceive it as a distinct phenomenon. The minutes or hours of abnormal consciousness following the seizure are called the *postictal* period. The interval between seizures is the *interictal* period.

The aura. Automatic behavior or peculiar sensations often precede complex partial seizures and occur even though the person is alert (Box 1.8). He abruptly feels compelled to make some type of movement, such as turning his head to the right or left or demanding, pouring, or drinking water. Chewing movements,

---

Box 1.8
Common auras in complex
partial epilepsy

Upset stomach or nausea

Urgent need to defecate

Unpleasant smells or tastes

Auditory or visual hallucinations

Automatic behavior sequences

Depersonalization

Intense fear

Déjà vu

Jamais vu

---

lip-smacking, spitting, or grimacing are part of the aura for some individuals, although these automatic movements also may appear during the seizure proper. Such embarrassing automatic activities as undressing and urinating occasionally occur. Often a person with complex partial epilepsy will recognize the familiar ritual and may announce that he is going to have a seizure.[12]

With the "uncinate" form of complex partial seizures, the patient senses and often complains of a disagreeable smell or taste. The name refers to the uncus of the temporal lobe, a part of the brain which was once considered important in the perception of odors. Complaints of nausea and abdominal cramps are fairly common in uncinate fits and may lead to vomiting, sweating, and pallor. Auras that involve peculiar smells or tastes have slightly more significance than other auras because they are often a sign of a tumor in the temporal lobe of the brain.[13]

Auditory hallucinations also occur in some auras. These usually consist of music or a buzzing sound, but occasionally they are more menacing and involve threatening voices. Visual hallucinations occur less frequently than auditory hallucinations. Even less common—but sometimes reported—are feelings of depersonalization and paranoid ideas. With depersonalization, the patient feels separated from his body. Victims of this delusion feel as if they are watching their soulless bodies go through activities in which they are not involved. Other psychiatric complaints include feelings that they are being persecuted by friends, family, and strangers and that remarks and activities occurring around them are actually referring to them. The person with these delusions feels that all the world is involved in a conspiracy against him. Some patients have attacks of intense, groundless fear. These psychiatric symptoms contribute to these patients' occasionally being misdiagnosed as schizophrenic.[14]

Also characteristic of some complex partial auras are feelings of intense familiarity with events just occurring (*déjà vu*) or total unfamiliarity with events that have occurred many times before (*jamais vu*). These are not abnormal feelings—many people without neurologic problems experience them from time to time—but their association with seizures makes them helpful indicators of an impending seizure.[15]

Abnormal electrical discharges detected by the electroencephalograph are usually just as prominent during the aura as during the seizure proper, but the patient perceives the two stages quite differently. The seizure victim can usually describe the aura vividly and in considerable detail, even while it is occurring. After the seizure is over, the affected person usually remembers the aura but has no memory of the ictus. Occasionally the aura occurs without any other seizure activity. This simply means that the spread of abnormal electrical activity has not followed the pattern usually involved in a conventional attack. Auras occur with other partial or generalized seizures, but they are most complex with complex partial (psychomotor) seizures.

The ictus. The seizure proper or ictus in complex partial epilepsy may be just a prolonged staring spell or may evolve into a generalized tonic-clonic (grand mal) seizure. Fairly complicated but pointless behavior such as running, laughing, or crying may occur. The patient may wander aimlessly, speak in unintelligible phrases, drink water, go to the bathroom to urinate or defecate, or simply hide. Rarely, patients appear to have sexual climax during the seizure; this phenomenon is most common in patients with seizures triggered by sexual excitement.[16]

During the ictus, which lasts seconds or minutes, the patient loses consciousness or has a profoundly altered state of consciousness. He will remember little or none of the episode when he has recovered from the seizure. The ictus is usually not associated with incontinence, tongue-biting, or tonic-clonic muscle activity unless the episode progresses to a generalized seizure.

With especially brief seizures, the patient may be completely unaware that a seizure has occurred. These absence attacks resemble petit mal epilepsy, but the electroencephalogram will not show the typical three-per-second spike-and-wave pattern of petit mal. Psychomotor absence attacks often occur coincidentally with other types of complex partial seizures, and with many types of complex partial seizures the duration of altered consciousness may vary dramatically from one episode to the next.

The postictal period. The interval between the seizure proper and the return to normal consciousness and function lasts two to ten minutes in most cases and is characterized by disorientation, inattention, and limited activity. Patients with psychomotor seizures that evolve into generalized seizures may become very irritable during this confused period, sometimes injuring themselves or those about them. Fortunately, postictal violence or anger is uncommon, and those few who exhibit it usually do not remember their behavior when the postictal confusion ends. This behavior is seen in both men and women.[17]

Rarely, patients undress and act sexually provocative during the postictal period, but the behavior is easily recognized as purposeless. As the postictal confusion clears, some patients experience sexual arousal, making the postictal behavior seem more purposeful than it actually was. This occurs too infrequently to be sure that one sex is more susceptible than the other, but most of the few instances described have involved women.[18]

The interictal state. The interval between unequivocal seizure episodes is called the interictal period. During this time the patient should be free of all seizure phenomena. At least in some patients with complex partial seizures, psychologic problems may be obvious even during the interictal period. Personality traits and psychologic disturbances of the interictal period that were not evident before or soon after the appearance of the seizure disorder may become very disruptive for the patient and his family after years of seizure activity.[19] These interictal complications are considered in detail in the next chapter and in Chapter 9.

FOCAL MOTOR, FOCAL SENSORY, AND JACKSONIAN SEIZURES. Focal seizures are partial seizures that affect movement or sensation in a limited area of the body. Evidence of the seizure may be nothing more than recurrent numbness in an arm or jerking of a leg (Box 1.9). If the abnormality is this limited, the patient is

---

Box 1.9
Features of Simple Partial Seizures
(Focal Motor or Focal Sensory)

Little or no warning of impending seizure

Electroencephalogram abnormal in
limited distribution

Focal limb movement in focal motor

Sequential muscle contractions with
jacksonian seizure

Focal numbness, burning, or tingling with
focal sensory

No loss of consciousness

No postictal confusion

---

said to have focal motor or focal sensory epilepsy, and the symptoms occurring are called elementary or simple. During these elementary partial seizures, the patient usually remains entirely alert, even if part of a limb or an entire limb has rhythmical involuntary contractions. Some focal sensory seizures involve vision or hearing. With this type of epilepsy the affected person may have transient episodes of peculiar vision or hearing. Visual phenomena may involve little more than flashing lights, and auditory complaints may include hearing menacing voices.

Seizures may start as simple or complex partial attacks and progress to generalized, grand mal attacks. In many types of epilepsy the secondary generalization may occur so rapidly that the seizures appear to be generalized tonic-clonic episodes until electrical studies of the brain reveal the progressive spread of abnormal activity throughout the outer layers of the brain. If the progression occurs over seconds rather than milliseconds, the progression from a focal to a generalized seizure will be more apparent, and the seizure may be called sequential rather than partial or generalized. Twitching in the thumb may spread to the arm and lead to a generalized tonic-clonic convulsion in what is called a jacksonian "march" or jacksonian seizure (after Hughlings Jackson, a neurologist who studied this type of sequential seizure activity).[20]

Simple partial epilepsy is especially easy to misdiagnose. Complaints of illusory flashing lights may be ascribed to eye disease, and the perception of a "crawling" or pins-and-needles sensation over an arm may be ascribed to injuries to a nerve in the affected limb. Because transient focal motor activity is often confused with a movement disorder and focal sensory activity is difficult to establish objectively, this type of seizure activity is often recognized only after it has been a problem for a long time. If the focal seizure becomes more generalized, the nature of the problem usually becomes obvious.

Alternatively, more progressive nervous system disorders may be misdiagnosed as partial epilepsy. Movement disorders are found in Huntington disease, Parkinson disease, and other degenerative diseases of the brain. The common migraine headache can give the illusion of flashing lights and other peculiar sensory phenomena. A twitching arm or a posturing leg caused by the early onset of Huntington disease may be misconstrued as restlessness in a child.

One form of focal epilepsy, called "benign focal epilepsy of childhood" or Rolandic seizures, almost always disappears as the child matures. Mid-temporal central spikes, that is, spikes around the central (Rolandic) fissure of the brain, are seen on the electroencephalogram, most often during sleep. The seizures are occasionally generalized and are also most likely to occur during sleep. These seizures are easily controlled with antiepileptic drugs and stop by the end of adolescence.[21]

Epilepsy is a family of disorders. All members of the family exhibit abnormal nerve-cell activity in the brain, but the spectrum of complaints and phenomena associated with epilepsy is enormous. What is most commonly recognized as epilepsy is the generalized tonic-clonic seizure disorder. What is most often not recognized as epilepsy is the generalized nonconvulsive or absence seizure disorder. Regardless of what type of epilepsy a patient has, his epilepsy makes him the victim of prejudices and misconceptions that have only recently exhibited signs of abating. Generalizations about intellectual and emotional characteristics of people with epilepsy are inappropriate and usually inaccurate. Most types of epilepsy do not disturb the affected person's ability or desire to live and work in conventional ways. Especially in patients with idiopathic epilepsy who take medication, the true limitations imposed by the disorder may be negligible.

Chapter 2

The Adult
with Epilepsy

Personal and family problems caused by epilepsy in an adult vary from the negligible to the devastating. With effective anticonvulsant treatment, many adults with epilepsy face virtually no limitations on their daily routines and long-term goals. The individuals least disturbed by the disorder are those with no apparent seizure activity, who take their daily medication and suffer no adverse side-effects. For this group, work, recreation, sexual activity, and family interactions proceed normally, largely undisturbed by the threat of seizures.

Unfortunately, this ideal is infrequently achieved. Complete control of seizures and persistent tolerance of anticonvulsant medication are often elusive. Most adults with epilepsy are uncomfortably aware of their neurologic disorder, and it affects many aspects of their lives.

Social Adjustment

Adjusting to epilepsy means working, relaxing, and striving for personal goals with as much success as the average person without a seizure disorder. How well an individual copes with epilepsy is closely related to how well controlled the seizures are. Advances in treatment have been dramatic over the past few decades and promise to be equally substantial in the near future, but these developments cannot eliminate the fear and pessimism that often burden individuals with poorly controlled seizures.[1]

The type of seizure a patient has plays an important role in determining whether the patient can achieve a relatively normal lifestyle. The least disruptive types allow the most normal lifestyles. Social adjustment is normal in 87 percent of patients with nonconvulsive absence seizures, regardless of their other problems. Individuals with generalized tonic-clonic (grand mal) seizures that develop because of head injury, brain tumor, or encephalitis have, not surprisingly, poor social adjustment.

Intellectual problems, personality disorders, and other handicaps that occasionally appear in people with epilepsy make adjustment more difficult. Large studies of social adjustment have found virtually normal lifestyles in 92 percent of patients whose seizures are not associated with any intellectual or personality disorders. These people are not free of substantial problems, but the social obstacles they face are surmountable. Even with personality disorders, as many as 52 percent of people with epilepsy have a normal social adjustment. Intellectual impairment reduces this fraction to 21 percent, and a combination of intellectual and personality disorders reduces it to 15 percent.[2]

An important element in any social adjustment is to set reasonable goals. The physician can help the epileptic patient and his family set realistic goals by providing an assessment of the patient's limitations and capacities. What is feasible will be determined in large part by the patient's intellectual abilities, personality traits, and seizure control. An accurate appraisal of what is possible will help the patient to realize his potential and will cut down on family pressure to achieve unreasonable goals.

The physician can also anticipate problems and suggest strategies to help the patient circumvent them. Unfortunately, many patients consider their doctor as just another reminder of the epilepsy and tend to avoid consulting him. Manageable problems, such as impotence caused by an anticonvulsant, mood swings as seizure control improves, and injuries suffered during seizures, may go unresolved because of the patient's reticence and pessimism. But of course even the most concerned physician cannot supply the daily encouragement and support that patients need. The real burden of helping a person adjust to epilepsy falls on the family.

Guilt

One of the more paradoxical adjustment problems faced by people with epilepsy is coping with guilt. Many victims of seizure disorders feel personally responsible for their predicament. This is especially true of accident victims, even when they were nothing more than innocent bystanders. "If only I'd been more careful" is a common refrain among those who have suffered head trauma leading to epilepsy. The combination of this sense of responsibility and a feeling of worthlessness that often develops if seizures limit the person's activities can lead to depression and self-destructive behavior.

Many adults with epilepsy feel guilty about the impact their disorder has on other family members. "What will it do to my family?" was the central concern of one man whose business career ended when his seizures began to interfere with his memory. Another young man who was already totally disabled by arthritis and heart disease expressed the same concern even though he had no job to lose. He explained, "The kids looking at you, it upsets you." His father had already had two heart attacks, and he was afraid that seeing him have a seizure might bring on another heart attack. The distress they have brought to their families is a common theme in discussions with patients whose seizures are poorly controlled.

Family and friends inadvertently or purposely reinforce such guilt feelings when they insist that the person with epilepsy brings on the seizures by not taking appropriate measures to prevent them. The wife of a middle-aged man with idiopathic seizures that began when he was about forty years old insisted that his seizures would not occur so often if he would eat a low-fat diet. Her admonitions were well-intentioned, but they intensified her husband's suspicion that he was to blame for the seizures that plagued him.

Aggravating these feelings of guilt is the embarrassment that comes with each epileptic attack. When the seizure occurs in public, many patients feel ashamed. One young man with complex partial (psychomotor) seizures explained, "You sit up at night wondering if you should apologize, but you think, 'What are you apologizing for, for falling down and being sick?' I've reached the point where I don't give a damn what people think."

Being indifferent to the reactions of family, friends, and strangers is difficult, perhaps impossible. The physician often has limited contact with the patient's family and friends, and so has little opportunity to discuss the causes and management of the disorder with them. By involving at least the immediate family in discussions with the physician, the patient can shift some of the burden of explanation to the doctor. Both the individual and the family must recognize that a person with seizures has no more reason to feel guilt or shame than the victim of a stroke or a heart attack.

Isolation

Whether out of embarrassment, guilt or weariness at having to explain their seizures, people with epilepsy often withdraw from family, friends, and colleagues. All too often these groups allow or encourage this alienation because of their own discomfort with the seizure disorder. Those relationships which do not dissolve often change dramatically. Even if these surviving relationships are not fragile, the person with epilepsy routinely shelters them from anger, abuse, or even assertiveness. The relationship with a physician will not be tested unless the patient develops a self-destructive bent. Dependence upon a spouse may be so extreme that the patient surrenders virtually all autonomy. The epileptic individuals' real or imagined loss of independence may eventually breed antagonism toward those they are dependent upon, and this anger increases their isolation from friends and colleagues.

In many cases the family isolates the epileptic member from normal family stresses out of concern that agitation will bring on a seizure. In fact, although emotional incidents may trigger seizure activity, they usually play a relatively minor role. Identifying situations that seem to trigger seizures is one valuable measure to pursue, but attempting to eliminate emotional stress from the patient's environment is usually more disruptive and disturbing than the stress itself. Trying to protect the person with epilepsy from emotional strain isolates him from the social activities and discussions that are part of a normal family life.[3]

The Sick Role

The family that designates a person with epilepsy as "sick" suspends that person's normal social responsibilities, such as providing income, assistance, and comfort to the family. In the most extreme cases, the individual with seizures is not even expected to "pull himself together." A person with any illness, whether it be acute or chronic, routinely regresses, at least temporarily, and becomes dependent upon family and friends. Unfortunately, denial of abilities, as well as of disabilities, may be part of the patient's reaction to a neurologic disorder.[4]

Ideally, a sick person should want to get better and should seek competent help in the struggle to recover. This ideal is not met by the family that relies upon the disabilities of the individual with epilepsy—whether they be real, contrived, or imposed—to explain family problems or to provide income from disability checks. The family may explicitly tell the patient that the neurologic problem is totally disabling and that recovery is impossible even when that is far from true.

The physician caring for the person designated "sick" may face considerable resentment if he considers the individual with epilepsy less disabled than the family thinks he is. In such situations it may be less important to make an accurate assessment of the patient's abilities and prognosis than to give the family a practical strategy for allowing the patient out of the sick role. The physician must ascertain why the patient was allowed or obliged to assume this dependent role in the first place and what purpose is served by his remaining in it. If what is needed is a steady flow of disability checks to support the family, then real work options must be found for the patient or for other members of the family. If an unstable marriage is being held together by the demands of an all-consuming illness, then the instability of the marriage must be dealt with.

Rehabilitation

Life is very different after a person develops seizures, and rehabilitation is often appropriate. An executive who develops epilepsy after an automobile accident may lose both her job and her pride. A person whose entire self-image has been caught up in work may sink into a paralyzing depression. Rehabilitation must address both the possibility of employment and the need for self-esteem. Getting the patient involved in a group of people with similar types of epilepsy is often helpful. A group can dispel the feelings of isolation and hopelessness that often develop when a seizure disorder appears in adult life. Without some such intervention, the person with epilepsy is likely to become unassertive and isolated and to lose interest in work, social activities, and family life.[5]

Return to employment should not wait for control of the seizures. Individuals whose seizures are only partially controlled can and should work. Obviously, generalized convulsions that occur several times a day will drastically reduce a person's employability. Of the people with epilepsy who are unemployed, 70 percent have more than one seizure every six months and most have more than one seizure monthly. Only 50 percent of those who work have seizures this frequently. In fact, returning to some type of work may have an antiepileptic effect. People with seizure disorders who have regular employment exhibit fewer problems with seizure control than those who are idle.

Younger people tend to respond better to rehabilitation programs than older people, especially if epilepsy is their only neurologic problem. An early return to being self-supporting is also advantageous; individuals who are on welfare or other types of support when rehabilitation begins are much less likely ever to return to work than are patients who need to earn a living.

Employment

Twenty-one percent of adults with epilepsy believe that the greatest problem they face is securing and holding a job. According to employment statistics, the outlook is not as grim as these people suspect, but anyone with a seizure disorder does face numerous employment problems. Finding and keeping a job are most difficult for those with both epilepsy and intellectual impairment, especially if the epilepsy is not fully controlled. In fact, frequency and severity of seizures correlate best with difficulty obtaining and holding a job—a finding that suggests that real disability is a more important determinant of unemployment than social prejudice against individuals with epilepsy. When general unemployment levels in the economy are close to 3 or 4 percent, an adult with well-controlled seizures, a good education, and no other health problems has as good a chance of finding a job as an adult without epilepsy. (Unfortunately, this is true only if the individual does not mention epilepsy as a problem on the job application form.)[6]

When people with epilepsy apply for jobs, about 62 percent deny or do not mention the disorder. This obviously leaves these individuals vulnerable to dismissal if the seizure disorder is discovered after they have been on the job for days or years. This reluctance to be frank is understandable and quite reasonable, however: of people with epilepsy who have problems securing a job, more than 40 percent are turned away simply because they admit to having epilepsy, even though 79 percent of Americans say they believe people with epilepsy should be hired for jobs that do not present special risks for them.

One very talented economist recruited to work for a European government discovered that the final application form asked specifically about epilepsy and anticonvulsant medications. Although these forms were allegedly just a formality, each part of the application stated clearly that no appointment was final until the patient's health status was deemed to be "satisfactory." The bulk of the medical questionnaire focused on epilepsy and psychiatric illness. Implicit in the form was the notion that people with epilepsy and people with psychoses presented special risks to the government. This man's seizures were fully controlled with very little medication, but answering the questions honestly would have barred him from a job he had already been promised on the basis of his training and talent. Answering them dishonestly left him open to dismissal months or years later if the truth was discovered. Blatant and inappropriate discrimination was being practiced, but the discrimination had been legislated by the government for which he planned to work.

Of those people who do indicate on job applications that they have a seizure disorder, about 25 percent of the employable ones are unable to find work even when the employment figures for the general population are at their best. When general unemployment is high, people who tell potential employers about their epilepsy face systematic exclusion from the work force. One 17-year-old girl with fully controlled seizures could not get job interviews for even the most unskilled work. Her mother investigated the problem and uncovered a consistent reluctance on the part of employers to risk hiring a young person with epilepsy. As recently as ten years ago, only one in eight employers would hire a person who admitted to having a seizure disorder. The level of acceptance has edged up slightly over the past decade, but epilepsy is still a formidable disadvantage in the job market.

Even patients with long-standing employment frequently report forced retirement or imposed disability leave because of their epilepsy. Of those who lose their jobs, about 30 percent are fired after having seizures at work. Many different types of employers routinely force people with epilepsy out of their jobs: hospital workers, law enforcement officers, and corporate managers who develop epilepsy all face pressure to give up their jobs. The concerns voiced by these employers are similar. They believe that people with epilepsy are accident-prone, that most work is too hazardous for them, that they require facilities to manage seizures on the job, and that seizures occurring on the job not only cut down on the productivity of the person with epilepsy but also disrupt the work of fellow employees and place those employees in danger. Although all of these assumptions are refuted by work statistics, many employers simply fall back on the observation that seeing someone have a seizure at work frightens co-workers.

Absenteeism, injuries, and job performance are about the same for adults with epilepsy as for adults without epilepsy. There is a difference in some industries, such as manufacturing: individuals with epilepsy perform slightly *better* than individuals with no chronic health problems. Obviously, epilepsy does impose restrictions on certain types of employment. A person who has frequent grand mal seizures cannot safely operate a tractor, for example. The better-than-average safety on the job found in most studies of adults with epilepsy probably reflects the common sense exercised by these people. Thirty-seven percent of adults with seizure disorders claim that their choice of work was influenced by their disorder.

Hospitalization

When seizure control is very poor, hospitalization may be required to allow the physician to investigate the poor control and to make dramatic changes in antiepileptic medications. Unfortunately, frequent hospitalizations disrupt work, education, and family life; and yet hospitalization rates for all types of epilepsies have shown a general increase over recent years. As people with epilepsy get older, they are hospitalized more frequently for problems related to their seizure disorders, such as aspiration and injuries. Women have been hospitalized at a consistently greater rate than men, by a factor of about 7 percent, over the past several years. This difference undoubtedly reflects a variety of social factors, since the types of epilepsy and the severity of problems faced by the two sexes are not significantly different. These social factors probably include the more limited repercussions of hospitalizing a person who does not work outside the home, as opposed to taking a person away from a job. With changing patterns of employment and decisionmaking in the family, this disparity between male and female hospitalizations may soon disappear.[7]

Hospitalization to reduce seizures is inadvisable unless a strenuous effort to control them in a normal environment has failed. The decreased stress, increased structure, and limited activity that are a routine part of hospitalization may reduce seizure activity without any alterations in antiepileptic medication. But the benefits of this artificial environment disappear as soon as the patient is discharged. What must be achieved is seizure control in the patient's usual environment. This may require altering that environment, such as eliminating flash photography from the vicinity of a person whose seizures are triggered by flashing lights, or simply adjusting medication until the patient can tolerate the routine stresses of home and work without having seizures (see Box 2.1).

Accusations of Malingering

As with any chronic disease, the person suffering from epilepsy has the option of exploiting it. Relatively minor problems with seizure control may be elaborated upon to gain sympathy, power, or freedom from responsibilities. In fact, exploitation of the neurologic disorder is unusual in adults, though it is often suspected by family members who cannot believe that a long-term problem could be out of the victim's control.

Box 2.1
Factors Lowering the Seizure Threshold

Common

Sleep deprivation
Alcohol withdrawal
Dehydration
Malnutrition
Systemic infection
Trauma

Occasional

Barbiturate withdrawal
Hyperventilation
Flashing lights

Rare

Specific noises
Reading
Sexual activity
Eating

Sometimes people with epilepsy are obliged to convince their families or co-workers that they truly do have a problem. Seizure disorders are so different from other chronic illnesses that patients and their families often suspect they are psychiatric disorders. Even when the family accepts the disorder as authentic, the person with epilepsy may feel obliged to convince them repeatedly of its severity. Resentment often develops within the family if the person with the chronic problem is perceived as an opportunist.

A rift developed between a totally disabled young man and his sister when he became eligible for social security because of his poorly controlled seizures. Although the young man had severe brain damage, and although his sister had been a good friend until the onset of the seizures, she did not believe that he was actually disabled and accused him of getting a "free ride" because he was "lucky." An older man, forced to retire after he developed seizures from head injuries suffered in an automobile accident, faced repeated insinuations from friends and family that he was trying to build a strong case for litigation. His insistance that he was the victim of an accident was routinely greeted by skeptical remarks, and he became obsessed with proving that he was not a fraud.

Much of the reluctance to recognize a family member's disability derives from an unwillingness to admit that a real tragedy has occurred in the family. Suggestions that the epilepsy is a "clever" or "useful" way to get out of work or to get disability benefits understandably offend the person with seizures, even though such remarks may just reflect the anxiety of friends and family who do not want to believe that the person with epilepsy is impaired.

Explaining Altered Behavior

When a generalized tonic-clonic (grand mal) convulsion occurs, there is little to explain to even the most uninformed observers. The victim loses consciousness, may be injured, and is obviously confused after the most dramatic part of the incident. It is more difficult for the person with epilepsy to explain less obvious seizure phenomena, such as bedwetting, staring spells, disorientation, nonsensical remarks, and disturbed speech. If the person is determined to conceal the seizure disorder, then explaining this aberrant behavior becomes even more difficult.

Altered consciousness at an inopportune time can be devastating. A 50-year-old woman with recurrent psychomotor and focal motor seizures from a brain tumor had a psychomotor seizure while driving. When the police found her confused and uncooperative in the midst of a traffic jam, they assumed she was drunk and placed her under arrest. Too confused to follow their instructions to leave the car, she was handcuffed, forcibly removed, and booked for resisting arrest. She was injured in the struggle and lost several thousand dollars' worth of cash and checks that she was carrying to the bank. Wanting to conceal her disability, this woman did not wear identification indicating that she had a seizure disorder. Even with a physician's letter explaining her behavior, she was obliged to appear in court to answer the charges brought against her.

A patient with epilepsy and kidney disease faced a similar predicament when police found him in a postictal stupor. They mistook his multiple dialysis punctures for track marks from drug abuse and arrested him as a presumed drug addict. His indignation when he recovered from his seizure did little to convince the police that he was anything but an offensive addict. Pleas that his doctor, rather than his lawyer, be called finally gained him credibility.

Other patients, even those whose seizures are fully controlled, sometimes find themselves having to prove that an unfortunate incident was *not* caused by seizure activity. Louise, a 24-year-old woman with fully controlled generalized seizures, had her driver's license revoked after an accident. She was struck by a car that went through a red light and had witnesses to attest to where the fault lay, but the motor vehicle bureau demanded that she prove she was not having a seizure when the accident occurred. They asked for objective tests, such as an electroencephalogram, to document that she was seizure-free. Though no one at the scene held her responsible for the accident, the bureaucracy treated this incident as an accident involving a person with epilepsy, rather than as just an accident. Since a physician was not in the car with her at the time of the accident, no one could provide an authoritative statement that she had not been having a convulsion. An abnormal electroencephalogram would not have meant she was under poor seizure control, since people with epilepsy very often have abnormal electroencephalograms between seizures, even on a dose of medication that controls the seizures. In any case, the possibility of a normal electroencephalogram was completely eliminated by the extensive head injury the woman suffered during the accident. To make matters worse, the driver of the car that had run the red light, on learning that the motor vehicle bureau had suspended the woman's license, filed suit against her on the grounds that by driving with a seizure disorder she had recklessly endangered him.

These are admittedly gross examples of legal problems faced by people who develop altered behavior during a seizure, but they are certainly not rare. Much of the difficulty can be avoided if the affected person carries information about the seizure disorder in a conspicuous place, such as on a bracelet or necklace. A card listing seizure type and medications and carried along with identification provides more privacy but is more easily overlooked by nonmedical personnel.

Coincidental Problems

For many people, seizures are merely one facet of a disease of the nervous system that produces several disabilities. Over 75 percent of patients with seizure disorders show some intellectual, behavioral, or neurologic problem. Seizures may appear with mental retardation and clumsiness in victims of cerebral palsy or with paralysis and speech disorders in individuals who have suffered strokes. In fact, the epilepsy may be a relatively minor feature of the disease. The accident victim with paralysis of his right side may find his seizures little more than an annoyance in comparison to the disability wrought by his paralysis. All of the individual's problems must be considered if any profitable management of the disorder is to be achieved. A patient may be uncooperative with medical personnel in trying to suppress his seizures if he considers the seizures a minor problem in comparison with others that are being ignored.[8]

Paralysis

Transient weakness in a limb or in an entire side of the body, a phenomenon called postictal or Todd's paralysis, occasionally develops after a seizure. The weakness rarely lasts more than a few minutes, but in some cases it lasts as long as 24 hours. Even brief weakness can be disabling if the patient's work demands a constant level of physical performance, such as is the case for a machine operator. Regardless of its duration, Todd's paralysis is not very common. What is much more common is the association of seizures with paralysis that develops after structural damage to the brain from trauma, stroke, or tumor. When a person has had epilepsy for several years and then develops weakness or clumsiness on one side, an unsuspected tumor or vascular malformation is probably responsible for both problems.

Dementia

About 15 percent of all people with seizure disorders are intellectually impaired. The impairment, which varies from slight memory disturbance to profound mental retardation, may be the person's principal difficulty. Fully 60 percent of the mentally retarded have some type of seizure disorder. It is probably through equating these dependent individuals with epileptic individuals in general that many of the common misconceptions about epilepsy arose. Epilepsy does not cause dementia (that is, impaired intellectual function), but some causes of dementia also cause epilepsy.[9]

Several types of seizure disorders are routinely associated with memory problems. Patients with complex partial (psychomotor) seizures frequently complain that they are not remembering new information as well as they did in the past. The wife of a 52-year-old security officer who developed psychomotor seizures in middle age complained that he repeatedly hid bank books and other valuables and then forgot where he had put them. He also had trouble calculating change and keeping track of cash. Because the epilepsy had already substantially restricted his activities, the family was reluctant to take his financial responsibilities away from him. All that was achieved by this consideration was increasing financial hardship for the entire family and growing anger at the man's incompetence. Rather than allowing resources to be lost because of her husband's memory disorder, the wife could have (and ultimately did) resolved the situation by taking all financial matters out of her husband's hands and accepting his anger and sadness at this further loss.

Prognosis

Both the adult with epilepsy and family members affected by the disorder worry about the long-term outlook. Insurance companies tell them that epilepsy increases the risk of early death, and friends tell of other people who were seizure-free after a few months of special diets, chiropracty, acupuncture, or other fads. The outlook, in fact, closely depends on the specific type of epilepsy a person has and the other health problems associated with it. Generalizations are difficult to make and unreliable for individuals to depend upon for long-term planning.

Remission

Remission is the disappearance of all seizure activity in a person with a history of epilepsy who is no longer on any anticonvulsant medication. Seizures that develop in or persist into adult life do not usually remit. This is especially true for individuals with abnormal electrical activity arising in the anterior temporal lobes. Not only will the complex partial seizures associated with these temporal lobe disorders require medication for decades, but even with the medication the seizures are often poorly controlled. Adults with any type of epilepsy are usually obliged to take antiepileptic drugs for the rest of their lives. Why seizures sometimes remit in children as they mature, but not in adults as they age, is unknown.[10]

Adults who have remained seizure-free on anticonvulsants for several years are often eager to stop taking the drugs. It is not easy to tell how long an interval free of seizures is adequate before the patient can safely give up the medication. Some patients free of seizures for four years will remain asymptomatic for life, and others free of seizures for ten years will have a convulsion within a week of stopping the medication. The usefulness of monitoring changes in the electroencephalogram to help decide when or if medication should be stopped is controversial. In children, brain-wave abnormalities are currently not considered a good reason for continuing antiepileptic medications in a child who has been seizure-free for several years. In adults, the relationship between the brain-wave patterns and the likelihood of recurrent seizures after years without seizure activity is unclear and very controversial. Most physicians do agree that if no structural lesion is evident in the brain and the electroencephalogram is normal after several years free of seizures, withdrawal of the antiepileptic medication can be attempted cautiously. This attempt should be made, of course, only if it is what the patient wants. A person with a history of epilepsy must be aware that the seizures may recur when the medication is stopped.

Mortality

Premature death caused by the seizure disorder is a common fear. Although mortality statistics lend some support to this fear, the premature deaths that do occur among people with epilepsy are generally not caused by seizure activity in itself. The ratio of observed to expected deaths for people with epilepsy is 2.3; that is, a patient is more than twice as likely to die at his current age than an identical person without epilepsy. But this mortality rate includes individuals who have seizures because of incurable brain tumors, massive head trauma, or fatal strokes. It is also inflated by the inclusion of children who succumb to congenital neurologic damage, accidental head trauma, or infantile brain tumors that caused the seizure disorder. In fact, if all patients with ascertainable causes of epilepsy are excluded from the mortality statistics, the mortality for people with idiopathic epilepsy is close to that of the general population. There is little, if any, increased mortality in people with idiopathic generalized absence (petit mal) seizures or complex partial (psychomotor) seizures, especially if seizures first appeared in adolescence and the person is female. There is no increased risk of early death in individuals with the benign Rolandic epilepsy of childhood. As would be expected in any condition that increases the risk of accidental injury, the observed increases in mortality rates are related to the severity of the seizure activity (see Box 2.2).[11]

Transient fluctuations in mortality rates occur. During the first two years after a person's first seizure, even if it is the only seizure ever observed, mortality is more than twice the expected rate. Because this increased mortality is largely a product of lethal conditions that cause the seizures, individuals with only one seizure have normal mortality rates if they survive these first two years. Mortality also shows a sharp increase for the interval 20–29 years after the initial diagnosis of the seizure disorder, a phenomenon that remains unexplained by current views of epilepsy and antiepileptic treatment. Also unexplained is the appreciably lower long-term mortality rate for women,

---

**Box 2.2
Factors Minimizing Mortality**

Idiopathic basis for seizures

Petit mal or Psychomotor seizure type

Benign epilepsy of childhood seizure type

Good seizure control

Female sex

Seizure onset in adolescence

which is 1.6 over 30 years, as compared to that for men, which is about 2.1.

Certain types of seizures do have a poor prognosis. Myoclonic epilepsies increase the mortality rate more than fourfold during the first year after the appearance of the seizures. Myoclonic epilepsies are relatively uncommon, and many of the conditions responsible for these types of epilepsy are lethal metabolic diseases. Generalized tonic-clonic seizures are associated with an increase of three and a half times in mortality during the first year after seizure onset. But again, it is symptomatic, not idiopathic, epilepsy, that drives up the mortality rates in these conditions. Generalized tonic-clonic seizures, for example, may be caused by a viral encephalitis.

Except for obvious intracranial causes of seizure activity and early death, such as meningitis, brain tumors, and strokes, no natural causes of death are notably prevalent in epileptic populations. Accidents occurring during seizures are causes of death experienced only by people with epilepsy, but the causes of death common in the general population—accidents, atherosclerotic vascular disease, and cancer—are also common in individuals with epilepsy. Status epilepticus, in which the patient has repeated seizures without returning to normal consciousness, is occasionally lethal if medical attention and effective anticonvulsant treatment are not obtained soon after the appearance of the intractable seizures, but this is a relatively uncommon condition.

The one cause of death that is unrelated to seizure activity and is inordinately common for people with seizure disorders is suicide (see Chapter 9). Accidents cause 5 to 16 percent of the deaths in individuals with epilepsy, but it can rarely be ascertained whether a seizure caused the accident. It is also unfair to blame antiepileptic drugs for the higher-than-expected incidence of accidents; excessive doses of such drugs may cause mildly impaired coordination and slow response times, but the most frequently lethal accidents, such as drownings, do not suggest that such problems play a major role. Some studies have suggested that anticonvulsant drugs decrease mortality by protecting against heart disease, but long-term mortality figures have not borne out this early impression.

Adults with epilepsy and their families often face social and medical problems because of the neurologic disorder, but these problems are surmountable if they are approached with flexibility and patience. In most cases, it is the patient with frequent seizures who has the most difficulty adjusting to his disorder, maintaining a normal family life, and holding a job, but even adults with infrequent or easily controlled seizures may be deeply affected by the need to deal with epilepsy as a daily concern. Most people with seizures can achieve a productive and satisfying lifestyle, but achieving that lifestyle may take considerable cooperation from family and friends. Common emotional reactions to the disorder, such as feelings of guilt and embarrassment, may incline the epileptic adult to withdraw from friends and relatives. Such withdrawal should not be allowed to end friendships and family ties.

Epilepsy usually can be adequately controlled so that it intrudes rarely, if ever, into the affected person's daily routine. Family and friends should be encouraged to treat it as an occasional inconvenience rather than as a perpetual tragedy. The adult with epilepsy never profits from being regarded as a functional cripple. Any family that treats the epileptic person as totally dependent should examine its motives for doing so. Even those people who face major restrictions on their activities because of the seizures or other nervous system problems associated with the seizures generally can and should develop lifestyles that maximize their independence and self-esteem.

Becoming and staying employed often plays a major role in this adjustment to the disorder. If familiar patterns of work become impractical because of the epilepsy, the patient must be willing to make job or career changes. Inactivity is demoralizing, and therefore dangerous; patients who must give up old employment goals must be encouraged to set aside their pride and any delusions they might have about miraculously returning to their old jobs, and to find new jobs that fit their changed abilities. If the patient has neurologic problems in addition to seizures, these must be addressed with rehabilitation or medication. They never justify allowing the patient to become totally inactive and dependent.

Chapter 3

Marital Problems

If a person with epilepsy is married, many of the problems caused by the seizure disorder will affect the other partner in the marriage. The problems that develop may be economic and social as well as medical. Until a few decades ago, the appearance of epilepsy in a man threatened the economic survival of his family. With an increasing number of women working outside the home, a husband's seizures do not carry such grave economic consequences, but now a wife's seizures may also change the couple's standard of living. When both partners contribute to the family income, a work disability in either will affect the living standard of both. Of course, the spouse of an individual with epilepsy may lose a reliable partner in more than just economic terms. Childrearing, housekeeping, socializing, entertaining, sexual initiative, and other elements of the marriage must be redistributed, especially when the person's seizures are poorly controlled.

If seizures are well controlled, the epilepsy may have little impact on either partner. But this is often not the case. The spouse without epilepsy becomes responsible for sustaining the family in many respects and may become overresponsible. A reasonable level of concern for and supervision of the partner with epilepsy may progress to an obsession with and surveillance of that partner. The best interest of the person with epilepsy is transformed into a long list of prohibitions. Violation of the prohibitions angers the spouse who enforces them, and enforcement irritates the spouse who is subject to them. Not surprisingly, this overresponsibility often leads to resentment in both partners.

Increased stress in the marriage results from the sexual problems that occasionally develop in individuals with seizures (see Chapter 4). The partner without epilepsy may turn elsewhere for sexual activity and companionship. Even if the marriage does not end in estrangement or divorce, it may deteriorate into much less than a partnership. The epilepsy may be blamed for any friction developing between spouses and may be used as a justification for excluding the affected spouse from decisions and activities that appropriately involve both.

Frequency of Marriage

Marriage is less common in individuals with epilepsy than in the general population. About 69 percent of all men and 70 percent of all women in the general population marry, but only 56 percent of men and 69 percent of women with epilepsy ever marry. Marriage patterns are more affected for men than for women, a disparity that perhaps reflects a significant difference in social attitudes toward men and women. Men with seizures are considered less reliable providers than men without seizures. Until very recently a woman's ability to provide financial support played a small role in the choice of a wife by most American men; in contrast, a man's potential as a provider was an important consideration in choosing a husband.[1]

The age at which the seizure disorder first appears influences the likelihood of marriage for both sexes. If the first seizure occurs after age 20, the affected individual is as likely to be married or to get married as any member of the general population. Unfortunately, by age 20, 75 percent of the individuals who will develop epilepsy during their lifetime have already had their first seizure. The age at which complete seizure control is achieved also has an effect on marriage. For patients whose epilepsy is fully controlled by the time they are 12 years old, marriage is as likely as for the general population. Men with epilepsy who marry even though they have had poorly controlled seizures since childhood usually have marriages that end in early separation or divorce.[2]

Social factors probably influence these rates of marriage. Men have traditionally taken a more active role than women in proposing and arranging marriage. The basic element reducing marriage rates in both men and women with epilepsy, especially epilepsy that begins at an early age, is probably a lack of initiative or assertiveness.

Common Fears

To bystanders, generalized convulsions appear to be life-threatening. The first time a person sees his or her spouse have a grand mal seizure or a complex partial seizure that progresses to a grand mal seizure, he or she is likely to think the spouse is dying. Even if the nonepileptic partner knows that death during a seizure is unlikely, other fears linger. The wife of a man who had had more than one seizure a week for several years commented, "I always try to wake him up [when he has a seizure]. I'm always afraid he'll go into a coma." Even with well-controlled seizures there is the constant worry that the person with epilepsy will have a seizure while driving or near subway tracks or other dangerous locations. Family members often voice concerns about lethal accidents that can occur during seizures. Death, rather than additional disability, is the central fear.

Predictably, this fear is not often openly discussed between the two concerned parties. A middle-aged wife who was very outspoken in family group meetings about the dangers surrounding her husband because of his epilepsy admitted, "In my house, we don't discuss it." The rationale for this seems to be that imagining the dangers is upsetting enough without compounding the fear by discussing it. Unfortunately, maintaining this silence usually proves to be a substantial burden for the spouse who does not have epilepsy. One of the major values of family group meetings, in which several families with epileptic members get together to talk about problems at home, is that they give the whole family a safe forum for discussing such fears. The opportunity to explore the fears often serves to defuse them.

Overresponsibility

Constant surveillance can become an obsession for the spouse of the person with epilepsy. "It's what we call the watchdog effect," explained a young man whose epilepsy had developed after brain surgery to remove a blood clot; "I sing in the shower loud enough so that she won't worry." The constant watching and worrying are a strain on both partners. One spouse admitted, "I try to think of other questions to ask besides, 'Are you all right?' . . . I can never relax." In discussing the possibility of her husband's being arrested because of his confusion and erratic behavior, one wife remarked, "If you get arrested, I'll let them keep you. I need a day off."

With many types of seizure disorders, such as frequent psychomotor seizures, simply remembering to take medication becomes a substantial chore. A man with poorly controlled seizures and frequent bouts of transient amnesia needed his wife to call his workplace everyday to remind him to take his drugs on schedule. Even with this assistance, he would sometimes take out his pills, pour a glass of water, drink the water, and forget to take the pills.

This surveillance fosters resentment. The wife of a man with complex partial seizures was understandably concerned whenever he deviated from his usual schedule. As she put it, "Even the dog got upset when he was late." Her husband's seizures produced a transient disorientation and amnesia that could last for minutes or hours. Just as understandably, he felt entitled to alter his routine occasionally just to provide himself with a little diversion. If his wife tried to find him when he made an unplanned stop on his way home, he became furious. Her anxiety deprived him of the independence he wanted, and she was fully aware of the difficulties this posed. "I'm afraid to take over everything," she explained. The possibility of completely depriving epileptic individuals of control over their own activities is very real.

Being the caretaker in this type of situation obviously carries little reward. Even helping the person with epilepsy maximize the coveted independence goes unacknowledged. Techniques developed to help with drug scheduling or safety measures are often credited to the epileptic person's own ingenuity, even when it is his or her spouse that provides the technique. Credit is not given where it is due. The debt is too pervasive to acknowledge. "I always have to be there to catch him," one wife explained, "and I get angry, and I think, 'Let him fall' . . . I tell him to go lie down and he doesn't, and then he has a seizure, and I get angry, because he could have been upstairs in bed." The epileptic spouse tries to assert control over the problem, rather than merely taking precautions. When his or her ability to control the seizures proves to be a delusion, the spouse who advised caution must deal with the consequences.

The spouse's tendency to take on excessive responsibility is especially annoying because it is a tangible reminder of the seizure disorder. One successful executive with seizures commented, "If I hear her say, 'Are you all right?' one more time, I'll scream . . . It's a constant reminder that I'm not well anymore." Unfortunately, the watchdog relationship focuses so much attention on the person with epilepsy that other members of the family, including the ever-vigilant spouse, may be neglected. The epileptic executive felt extremely guilty when his wife became ill. He felt that he had been ignoring her problems. He only noticed that there was something wrong with her when she stopped being so watchful of him. The person with epilepsy may resent the constant scrutiny and yet also fear that it will not be there. One young man with seizures who was constantly trying to elude his wife's surveillance admitted that if she stopped being oppressively watchful he would assume she had given up on him.

Much of the overresponsibility is a reaction to poorly controlled epilepsy. As with other problems, overresponsibility fades as an issue when the epilepsy is fully controlled. When seizure control cannot be achieved, the responsibility must be shared. Once again the people best equipped to help manage the problem are other families with similar problems. Contact with people in similar situations provides perspective, if not solutions. An issue, like the need to sing in the shower, that seems oppressive when the couple are alone at home quite often seems trivial when it is discussed in a family group meeting.

Loss of a Reliable Partner

The transformation that occurs with a seizure is transient, but the helplessness and haggardness that often appear with the seizure can be devastating to the spouse of the person with epilepsy. The husband of a young woman who developed frequent complex partial seizures abandoned all hope of having a real marriage. He had little physical contact with his wife and depended upon his mother-in-law to take care of her. A middle-aged woman whose husband developed epilepsy after more than 20 years of marriage described the day he had his first generalized convulsion: "When they took him out, they had an old man strapped in a chair. He was good for nothing. The doctors told me he was in limbo." Uncertainty over what the epileptic spouse will be able to do soon gives way to uncertainty over when the helplessness will recur. With antiepileptic treatment, many patients return to fully normal activities, but their spouses are left with the persistent image of someone active and able suddenly becoming dependent.

When seizure control is difficult to achieve, the problems are much greater. The seizure disorder and the anticonvulsant medication may combine to produce an inactive, often sedated, individual. One man in his fifties with recently acquired epilepsy had held two jobs for more than 20 years and had constantly painted and cleaned the house. After developing seizures he abruptly stopped working around the house. Frequent and protracted bouts of confusion forced him to retire from his jobs. His seizure control was poor despite antiepileptic medication, and he sat home everyday staring out the window and watching television. "He's getting into not doing all the things he used to do," his wife complained. "I know I have to give him more time, but he sits and does nothing. I can't take it. If you're going to die, die moving. Before the seizures, everything was automatically done. Before, I depended on him to do everything; now I do everything." The inactivity and loss of motivation that may accompany poorly controlled seizures are usually viewed as "giving up." The nonepileptic spouse feels obliged to push the epileptic spouse into activity, an obligation that often brings resentment with it. The wife of a young man with post-traumatic seizures was annoyed by his sudden loss of drive: "I say fight back. It's too bad they're sick, but you can't let them go to sleep."

Paradoxically, the spouse who feels the need to push the partner with epilepsy into a more active life is often the same spouse who resists his initiatives to do things that might bring on a seizure or place him at risk if he had a seizure. The woman who complained that her husband was no longer working around the house was horrified to find him climbing a ladder outside the house to paint windows. The young wife of the trauma victim spent uneasy hours every time he went off to coach a touch football team. Even though both of these projects were familiar and had been reasonable before these men developed their seizure disorders, they now posed unacceptable risks as far as the wives were concerned. When the trauma victim decided to fix a clogged gutter by climbing out onto the roof of the house, his wife became furious. She felt that so dangerous an activity was simply an expression of her husband's lack of "consideration." Risking injury was equated with denying responsibility for the family.

In fact, refusal to avoid excessive risks is sometimes irresponsible, if not intentionally self-destructive. A nightclub performer who had had grand mal seizures since childhood was seizure-free when she took anticonvulsants regularly and avoided sleep deprivation, but she rarely did either. Whenever she felt well, she skipped medications, dabbled in illicit drugs, drank large quantities of liquor, and partied late into the night. Such binges predictably provoked seizures, but neither her husband, her children, nor her parents could dissuade her. Their efforts to restrict her lifestyle only prompted more damaging behavior. She refused to be "limited" by her epilepsy.

Sheltering the person who has epilepsy may go well beyond reducing the risk of accidental injury. There is often an abiding fear that domestic problems will bring on a seizure, and so the person with epilepsy is often sheltered from day-to-day problems. Problems with the children or with finances are hidden. Excitement over parking tickets, unpaid bills, and school problems are all avoided. In many cases, the epileptic spouse feels bitter about being excluded from crises. One middle-aged man with complex partial seizures complained, "You're not even called upon to do what you're expected to do [as a parent and husband]. It's the same as saying, 'You're not capable and so we're not calling you.' " A younger man explained, "It's like being thrown in a closet."

The costs of maintaining a stable environment around the person with epilepsy include resentment in the protective partner and anger in the partner whose disability is emphasized by the protection offered. The nonepileptic spouse cannot voice resentment because of fear that the complaint will upset the delicate balance that spares the family the burden of recurrent seizures. The often outspoken complaints from the spouse with epilepsy that he or she is not being given a fair share of family responsibilities may compound the protective spouse's feelings of being misunderstood and unappreciated.

Isolation

Social isolation is as much a problem for the nonepileptic spouse as it is for the person with epilepsy. The wife of a man with unexplained seizures complained, "You find people are afraid of you. It's like you have something more than epilepsy, like the plague." Misconceptions and prejudices that seemed rather innocuous in family members and friends before the epilepsy developed become a source of constant annoyance and interference. Neighbors are often concerned that their children will be upset or even injured by seeing an epileptic attack. They may stop visiting a neighbor who has epilepsy. This causes special problems for couples with young children, because they face the same misconceptions when they try to get a babysitter. There is the concern that the individual with epilepsy will be erratic or violent or simply sick while the babysitter is there. This aversion to sickness is not unusual and not confined to epilepsy. But it is erroneous to believe that a person with epilepsy is likely to have a frightening or dangerous episode at any moment.

Social isolation extends even to near relatives. Like friends, family members may fear that a seizure will occur while they are around. Sheila, a young woman whose husband developed epilepsy within a few weeks of their marriage, found her mother's reaction at first confusing and then annoying. The mother had done volunteer work in hospitals and had never shunned the company of sick people. But when Sheila revealed that her husband had epilepsy, her mother stopped visiting their home and became remarkably unhelpful. When the couple had a child, the new grandmother refused to be in the house with the baby and its father unless Sheila was also there. Sheila thought her mother was intimidated by her husband's neurologic disorder. The older woman claimed that her main fear was that her son-in-law would hurt himself. Why this prevented her from spending more time with her daughter and grandson was never discussed.

Sheila's mother proved disruptive when a seizure actually did occur. Instead of trying to help, she screamed and cried. In her panic she left Sheila alone to deal with the seizure, forcing the couple's child to leave the room. The young boy, who had often seen his father have seizures and helped out by placing cushions around him, was more frightened by his grandmother's reaction to the seizure than by the seizure itself. In discussions with Sheila, her mother insisted that Sheila's husband was taking too much medication for his own good, but also that more must be done to eliminate his seizures.

Other members of the family were no more helpful than the mother-in-law. Visiting the homes of brothers and sisters became difficult for the couple because the family would not adjust to the epileptic man's needs. Even though his seizures were predictably triggered by flashing lights or watching television, when he visited his wife's family they all watched video games and television. At most extended-family activities, photographs were taken using flash attachments. This man with epilepsy was effectively excluded from most family activities simply because his relatives refused to alter their patterns of entertainment even slightly when he tried to participate.

Neighbors and friends may also be unhelpful or disruptive by offering useless advice. "They make you feel like you're doing something wrong," the wife of a man with seizures explained. "They ask if you've ever tried some medication they see mentioned on television." Much of the information provided through such channels is absurd, inaccurate, or simply banal, and explaining to a well-meaning friend or relative why the advice should not be followed can be a substantial chore. When the couple dismiss the advice as useless, the advising friend or relative often becomes offended. Intrusive friends or relatives do not realize that the couple are tired of having to deflect useless suggestions.

Even medically sophisticated people can be a burden. The wife of a young man with epilepsy was questioned by a nurse who elaborated on all the dangers the husband faced because of his seizure disorder. The young wife commented, "I want to leave when people start telling me what I should do. I'd like to say, 'Mind your own business. You couldn't possibly know what we know about it now.' " Doctors unfamiliar with her husband's case would tell her that she must be mistaken about details that she had repeated during more than a dozen hospital admissions. Her long and close association with her husband's illness made her much more sophisticated about the problem than the majority of the medical personnel she had to deal with, and perceiving this made her feel even more isolated.

Much of this feeling of isolation can be minimized by associating with people in similar situations. Most families with epileptic members do not realize that many other people face the same predicament. Once the feeling that this family problem is unique is dispelled, much of the fear and hopelessness can be eliminated. Discussions with others in similar dilemmas relieve the tension that inevitably develops in exchanges with unhelpful relatives and friends.

An additional problem faced by the spouse of a person with epilepsy is a feeling of isolation within the marriage. People with epilepsy often complain that their spouses are too intrusive, too watchful, too involved in their lives, but the spouses complain that the epileptic partners are constantly trying to exclude them from the problem that affects them both. The wife of a dialysis patient with poorly controlled partial and generalized seizures complained that her husband was most unwilling to discuss his seizures when they were at their worst. "Sometimes I try to talk to him," she explained, "but he says it's nothing." It seems that individuals with epilepsy do not want anybody to notice their seizures—even their husbands and wives. "He does not believe that he disturbs us," suggested the middle-aged wife of a man with complex partial seizures. "He thinks there is something wrong with me . . . not him." Even though the seizures are extremely disruptive in the lives of both partners, the spouse with epilepsy may resist involving his or her mate in managing them. One man who developed seizures after being involved in an automobile accident justified this desire to exclude his wife by claiming that her attention was condescending and even dictatorial. He explained, "I sense that she's always on the edge [of her chair]. She's always watching me." A more basic complaint is that involving the spouse in controlling the seizures deprives the epileptic individual of the little self-control and responsibility he still has.

The friction between marital partners grows when poor seizure control forces them to spend much stress-filled time together. If the epilepsy can be fully controlled, the friction subsides. If control of the epilepsy is elusive, then involvement of the couple with other couples who also face poorly controlled seizures may be helpful. Discussing the friction with people who really know what the problems are makes the issues between the spouses much less abrasive.

Separation and Divorce

The constant strain of dealing with epilepsy makes divorce a very real consideration. "At what point will I break?" asked the wife of a young man who developed seizures within weeks of their marriage. "I've never been married to a normal man." She could not help wondering what a relationship with a man unburdened with this problem would be like. The wife of a middle-aged man with complex partial seizures admitted, "I'm always screaming, 'Divorce!' . . . The worst part of it is when you go through a period of getting better." After hope develops that daily life can be fairly normal, the return of seizures is especially devastating.

Deception

When a person conceals his epilepsy from his spouse until months or years after they are married, the additional feeling of deception adds to the instability of the marriage. Many people believe that revealing their epilepsy will destroy their chances of marrying. Once they are married, revealing the problem will only serve to undermine their partners' trust. The deception is self-defeating. It leaves the epileptic individual with the feeling that his marriage can founder on one careless incident or remark. It denies the partner without epilepsy the opportunity to decide whether to accept responsibilities that are a part of the usual marriage contract.

When to discuss epilepsy is a dilemma for most people as they become emotionally or sexually involved with someone. It is awkward and usually considered socially inappropriate to discuss medical problems with casual acquaintances, but many intimate relationships start with casual acquaintance. If a long-term intimate relationship is likely, the partner who does not have epilepsy should be told of the disorder before dramatic changes in living arrangements are made. Epilepsy should be discussed in the same terms as any chronic medical problem, such as diabetes mellitus or rheumatoid arthritis. If the person with epilepsy is uncomfortable or uncertain of the facts, an informed and articulate health professional should be asked to help in the discussion. Rather than simply announcing "I have epilepsy" and waiting to see if the lover or suitor is terrified, a more reasonable approach is to say that a chronic problem involving the nervous system has been under treatment for some time and then to explain, or to allow a health professional to explain, exactly what the problems are. A concerned lover should not be intimidated by a problem that is already being managed. Taking the initiative in disclosing the disorder allows the person with epilepsy to develop a frank and relaxed intimacy.

Infidelity

The sexual problems that accompany poorly controlled epilepsy may deprive the nonepileptic spouse of a sexual partner. Infidelity is a natural consequence of such sexual deprivation (see Chapter 4), but how often it occurs is unknown.

Sexual problems can be used to disrupt the marriage. If the spouse without epilepsy turns to a sexual partner outside the marriage, this provides an excuse for ending the marriage. Infidelity is a more socially acceptable reason for divorce than an inability or unwillingness to cope with the problems of epilepsy. The spouse with epilepsy can feel simply wronged, rather than deserted, and the spouse without epilepsy can claim provocation for the infidelity. One or both partners may seize on the infidelity as an excuse to end an exhausting and unsatisfying relationship.

There is obviously no single approach to help ensure the stability of an intimate relationship. When a marriage shows signs of falling apart because of the strain of epilepsy, family counseling is appropriate. Group meetings of families with epileptic members can also be useful in this context. Insights on how to deal with specific marital problems emerge when a group of couples share their own techniques and failures. One woman who joined such a group expected her marriage to end within a year; she felt she had to leave her husband because he was incapable of coming to terms with his seizure disorder. After several months of meeting with other women in similar situations, she recognized that neither she *nor* her husband could accept his disorder and this insight, curiously, defused the problem for her. She had felt that she was a failure as a wife, but after talking to other equally frustrated wives she realized that it was the neurologic problem, not their own shortcomings, that was eroding all their marriages.

Epilepsy often puts strains on marriages and other intimate relationships, but it need not be the reason for ending these relationships. Both partners must first recognize what problems are being fostered by the seizure disorder and then look for techniques to minimize these problems. The nonepileptic partners often do not realize how much of the anger and resentment they feel derives from being overresponsible for the person with epilepsy. Allowing the epileptic partner to take charge of whatever he can reasonably do will reduce much of the friction in these relationships. The partners with epilepsy, in return, must not expose themselves or their families to excessive risks.

Sexual problems often arise when seizure control is poor, aggravating problems already facing the couple. Additional stress may come from friction with members of the family who perceive the epilepsy with fear or disbelief. All of these problems usually can be surmounted if the couple is able and willing to discuss them. Such discussions may not work well if they are limited to the affected couple, because neither partner can be objective. What usually does help is going to a family counselor or sex therapist, who can identify and resolve the difficulties.

Chapter 4

Sexual Activity

People with epilepsy face a higher than average risk of having sexual problems. They face the same problems and exhibit the same abnormalities found in the general population, but with a slightly higher frequency. In some cases the sexual dysfunction may be directly related to the epilepsy or its treatment, and in other cases the connection may be debatable. Sexual problems are as treatable in people with epilepsy as in people in general. Anticipating the problems that may develop and treating them aggressively will spare the epileptic individuals and their partners much frustration.

Risk of Sexual Dysfunction

The definition of "normal" sexual activity is becoming more and more inclusive as sexual practices in the general population come under closer scrutiny. When any group is subjected to long-term medical observation of sexual behavior, it is likely to seem that the members of that group have more sexual problems than "normal" people. In fact, people with epilepsy may have little, if any, more sexual difficulty than the general population; the more detailed information available on them may just highlight their difficulties.

With these qualifications in mind, one can fairly say that most people with epilepsy lead normal sex lives. But for certain individuals (such as those with complex partial seizures) and under certain circumstances (such as poor seizure control) sexual function is often adversely affected. In most instances, the main sexual dysfunction is a lack of interest, rather than an actual inability to perform. Fear that sexual intercourse or excitement will cause seizures may inhibit not only the individuals with epilepsy but their partners as well. Sexual eccentricities, such as transvestitism and fetishism, are rare in the population suffering from seizure disorders, but do occur in some people with complex partial epilepsy (see Box 4.1).

Controlling seizures will not eliminate all of these sexual problems. In fact, efforts to treat the seizures can cause problems of their own. Some people lose their sex drive as a side effect of antiepileptic medications. Others have distressing cosmetic problems with long-term use of antiepileptic drugs. Changes in appearance may undermine the patient's self-confidence, thus lessening sexual activity.

Established couples develop sexual inhibitions and anxieties primarily when seizure control is poor. The simplest, but often the most elusive, solution to this problem is improved seizure control. When that is not feasible, other ways must be found to minimize the disruptive effects of the epilepsy. Reticence is a

---

Box 4.1
Sexual Dysfunctions Described
in Individuals with Epilepsy

Hyposexuality

Transvestitism

Fetishism

Exhibitionism

"Sexual seizures"

Drug-related impotence

substantial barrier to the resolution of sexual problems: many patients are reluctant to discuss their sexual difficulties, and many physicians hesitate to ask detailed questions about sexual dysfunction. When the problem has been fully identified, it is more easily remedied.

Sexual Problems with Complex Partial Epilepsy

Many people with complex partial epilepsy experience sexual problems. Decreased sexual activity (that is, hyposexuality) is common in both men and women with this type of epilepsy. It is not simply a reaction to chronic illness: hyposexuality occurs in 50 percent of people with complex partial epilepsy, but in only 30 percent of people with other chronic medical disorders, including grand mal epilepsy. Hyposexuality is not properly a sexual complaint, since most individuals with complex partial epilepsy do not complain about their lack of interest in sex. If any complaints are offered, they usually come from the epileptic person's sexual partner.[1]

Impaired Libido

Lack of sexual interest, rather than ability, is primarily responsible for hyposexuality that often accompanies complex partial epilepsy. The men are not physiologically impotent, and the women do not have pain with intercourse; they simply lack interest in initiating sexual activity. Many people whose complex partial epilepsy started before puberty or at puberty remain without sexual experience throughout their lives. If the complex partial epilepsy starts later in life, after a sexual relationship has become established, the patient's partner will complain of a profound deterioration in sexual interest.[2]

Most individuals do not realize that the seizure disorder itself can affect sexual appetite. The patient often believes the anticonvulsant medication is responsible for a loss of libido; the patient's partner sometimes suspects that the patient is still sexually active, but with another person. Both of these conjectures are dangerous. The patient is tempted to stop the anticonvulsant medication to recover the lost libido, and the frustrated sexual partner doubts the patient's honesty.

The best that can be offered to the frustrated spouse is a frank assessment of the situation. The sexual appetite of the partner with complex partial seizures is not likely to return to its former level, though good seizure control sometimes helps. The spouse must decide whether this sexually unsatisfying relationship is gratifying enough in other ways to be worth continuing.

Sexual Eccentricities

Individuals with complex partial seizures also have more than the expected incidence of aberrant sexual behavior, such as fetishism, exhibitionism, and transvestitism. If the seizures begin in adulthood, eccentric sexual behavior may appear after years of more conventional sexual interests. The reason for this change is unknown. Sexual eccentricities are not part of seizure activity: the patient has no altered consciousness or loss of memory during the episode of sexual activity. Unusual sexual behavior usually occurs during the interictal period, the time when the patient is not having any apparent seizure activity.

A very few individuals, most of them women, do exhibit atypical sexual behavior during the aura or the seizure proper (ictus) of complex partial seizures. Stereotyped activities (automatisms) that occur may include undressing, masturbating, or attempting to stimulate other people. Behavior during these periods of altered consciousness may be in dramatic contrast to the individual's usual sexual behavior. One woman who was frigid between seizures became highly receptive during her seizures. Men with this type of sexual seizure occasionally have protracted erections (priapism), but they do not commit sexual attacks or other clearly purposeful sexual advances. Rape is not a feature of sexual seizures.[3]

Orgasm with Seizures

A few patients with complex partial seizures—again, almost all of them women—have orgasm as part of their seizures. In most of these women the orgasmic seizures occur premenstrually, and sexual satisfaction persists long after the seizure is over. When the orgasm occurs during the aura, the patient is able to recall enjoying it. Patients may be tempted to allow their seizure control to deteriorate in order to have these orgasmic seizures. Sometimes pleasurable sensations develop in the groin during the aura, accompanied by vaginal discharge characteristic of sexual excitation, but no orgasm follows. Sexual seizures have never been observed in prepubertal girls, and the few men who report changes in genital sensation with their seizures have unerotic or unpleasant sensations. For most women who have sexual seizures, the seizures seem to originate in the right temporal lobe. This is consistent with reports from neurosurgeons that stimulation deep in the temporal lobe occasionally elicits erotic feelings in women undergoing surgery to manage poorly controlled seizures.[4]

This type of sexual arousal may be more common than is reported, since most people do not volunteer information about their sexual feelings. If it *is* more common, then it may have substantial effects on individuals with complex partial seizures. In any case, the fact that these orgasmic phenomena occur almost exclusively in women suggests that seizures involving the temporal lobe affect sexual function in men and women quite differently. Sexual appetite and activity may be increased in some women with temporal lobe seizures. Even if a woman's sexual behavior changes only during the seizure itself, her exhibitionism, genital manipulation, and sexual receptivity may have considerable impact on her sexual partner. Whether her partner is indifferent, excited, or dismayed by this sexual display will have obvious consequences for their relationship.

Whether changes in sexual activity are transient phenomena or permanent side-effects of complex partial seizures is unresolved. So-called deviant sexual behavior is observed more often in patients with temporal lobe lesions developing before age 3 than in the general population. All that can be concluded from this observation is that people with early temporal lobe damage express different preferences from their peers. It may be that they simply give less inhibited answers to questionnaires about sex. Even when a patient's behavior is atypical for the social setting, it is difficult to consider the behavior pathological. A person appearing naked on a public beach or in a public park is considered an exhibitionist in some countries, whereas the same behavior is considered normal in other countries.

Other Causes of Poor Sexual Adjustment

A person with epilepsy may have sexual problems that are totally unrelated to the disorder. If a patient has impaired sexual function without impaired interest, the seizure disorder is probably not responsible for the dysfunction. All men with impotence (an inability to achieve or maintain an erection) and all women with dyspareunia (pain on intercourse) should be investigated for other possible causes.

The type of sexual dysfunction should always be considered. A man with complex partial seizures who has normal erections and ejaculations but feels no excitement at the time of orgasm is more likely to have a central nervous system problem associated with his epilepsy than a man who simply cannot have an erection. A woman who achieves no vaginal lubrication despite feeling considerable excitement at the time of intercourse should be investigated for a peripheral nerve or vaginal problem, even if she has poorly controlled seizures.

Occasionally, antiepileptic drugs are responsible for poor sexual performance, at least in men. Phenobarbital and primidone, which is partly converted to phenobarbital, are sometimes associated with impotence. When a patient has intact libido and no evidence of peripheral nerve damage to explain his impotence, a change in anticonvulsant medication is appropriate. Replacing phenobarbital with phenytoin or replacing primidone with carbamazepine may completely eliminate the sexual dysfunction.

Fear of Seizures During Sex

Sexual activity rarely triggers seizures. Nevertheless, if a seizure does occur during sexual intercourse, it can be devastating for both partners. People with epilepsy generally avoid activities that they believe will lead to seizures, whether that belief is based on observation or superstition. The fear of having a seizure can interfere with sexual enjoyment and can cause a couple to have sex less often. A seizure during lovemaking is often even more upsetting to the partner without epilepsy than to the epileptic partner. A person who first learns of his or her lover's seizure disorder in such a traumatic way may be an especially reluctant partner in the future.

One young woman always worried, during lovemaking, that the exertion of intercourse would cause her husband to have a seizure. This fear interfered with her ability to enjoy sex, and her extreme attention to his expression and movements made him too self-conscious to become fully aroused. He rarely ever reached orgasm despite sexual encounters that could last over an hour. The abnormal breathing pattern, the altered expression, and the stiffening of limbs that accompany sexual excitement in both men and women can resemble seizure phenomena, and this resemblance can make both partners too nervous to relax and allow excitement to lead to orgasm.

Overcoming this sexual inhibition is difficult even with the most uninhibited couples, but it is often impossible with couples who cannot talk frankly, or at least accurately, about their sexual problems and techniques. A counselor can assure the couple that a seizure during intercourse should not pose any special problems to either partner, and that seizure activity is no more dangerous during sex than at other times, but this reassurance may not dispel the worries of the partner without epilepsy. Both partners may find it terribly embarrassing to tell other people, even medical personnel, that the patient lost consciousness and had a seizure during lovemaking. Reassurance that this is an unlikely occurrence may do little to improve sexual performance or satisfaction.

Couples must be patient and committed if they are to overcome the inhibitions that develop when epilepsy is poorly controlled. Where considerable sexual dissatisfaction has developed, the couple should explore the possibility that a mutual tendency to withdraw from each other as a reaction to the epilepsy is making their sexual troubles more intense. Here again a family therapist can often help. Where there is little more to the sexual problem than anxiety, sexual therapy is often helpful.

Cosmetic Effects of Antiepileptic Drugs

Contributing to the social and sexual problems of young people with epilepsy are the cosmetic changes that often accompany antiepileptic therapy. The severe acne that characterized bromide treatment for seizures has become much less of a problem with the development of other anticonvulsants, but other commonly used drugs also cause skin changes. Phenytoin and, to a lesser extent, phenobarbital can cause coarsening of facial skin and darkening of facial hair. Arm and leg hair may also darken and appear thicker, but this is much less of a problem than facial hair for young women. Both men and women suffer from periodontal problems associated with phenytoin. Gingival hyperplasia, the overgrowth of the gums, is unattractive in either sex and often leads to loss of teeth unless patients submit to repeated gum surgery.

Effective treatment of these cosmetic problems is essential, at least in children and adolescents, because unless these side effects are controlled, patients may refuse to take their medication. Many people would rather risk occasional seizures than have gingival hyperplasia and lose their teeth. Changing medications may avoid further problems with skin, hair, and gums, but the existing changes will not disappear without some type of intervention. Gingival hyperplasia can be resolved with gum surgery (gingivectomy) and rigorous dental care. Hair on arms and legs may require shaving or chemical removal. Electrolysis is a better approach to facial hair, since it is more permanent and less likely to produce stubble.

Most people with epilepsy can and do have normal sex lives. There are specific problems that develop with certain types of seizures and with certain types of antiepileptic treatment, but most of these are surmountable. Some patients with longstanding complex partial epilepsy have little interest in sex, but even this symptom often abates with changes in seizure control or antiepileptic medication. Whenever sexual problems develop, the couple must recognize that the epilepsy or its treatment may be causing them. If the partners begin exchanging accusations or assume that the problem is untreatable before they seek remedies, both will suffer by the loss of the relationship.

Sexual dysfunctions are usually not caused by permanent changes in the sexual interests or abilities of the epileptic partner. Sexual activity can usually be restored to the way it was before the epilepsy if the sexual partners can frankly discuss the problems. A sex therapist or physician should be involved in the investigation and treatment of the sexual dysfunction. In many cases, all that is needed to correct the problem is a change of antiepileptic treatment, elimination of drugs used for conditions other than the epilepsy, or sexual counseling to minimize the inhibitions and fears the partners may have developed in response to the epilepsy.

Chapter 5

Childbearing and Inheritance

Separate from the sexual and marital problems associated with epilepsy are the concerns that develop when a couple thinks about having children. The decision about whether to have children is often affected by the frequency and severity of the seizures experienced by the epileptic spouse. The couple often wonders if their offspring will inherit a seizure disorder and if the parent with epilepsy will be able to care for the child. If it is the wife that has epilepsy, concern about birth defects from antiepileptic medications may dominate the couple's worries.

Reproductive Rates

Over the past thirty years, epilepsy has become less important in determining whether an individual has children, but it still plays a significant role. Certain problems more common in people with epilepsy than in the general population, such as severe mental retardation and other major handicaps, prevent some victims of epilepsy from having children. But even those without these obvious limitations have fewer children than do people in the general population (see Box 5.1).[1]

Reproductive rates are depressed for both men and women with epilepsy. Epileptic women who marry have only 69 percent as many liveborn children as do married women in the general population. Epileptic men who marry have as many children as the average married man, but fewer men with epilepsy marry.

Many factors influence this lower rate of reproduction. The specific type of seizure disorder seems to affect the reproductive rate, for example: as discussed in Chapter 4, complex partial epilepsy often decreases sexual interest. An epileptic woman who lacks sexual interest might marry for reasons other than sexual attraction, but she would probably have fewer pregnancies than women without epilepsy because she would avoid sexual intercourse. Overall, including those who never marry, women with complex partial epilepsy have an average of 1.64 children each, and men with this type of epilepsy have an average of 0.536 children each. These differences probably reflect differences in the rates of marriage for women and men with complex partial epilepsy.

Any statistics on reproduction must be interpreted with caution, because people do not always answer questions on such a

---

Box 5.1
Marriage and Reproduction

Men with epilepsy

Marry less often than women with epilepsy

Have less sexual interest than other men

Women with epilepsy

Have fewer children than men with epilepsy

Have fewer pregnancies than other women

Men and women with epilepsy

Marriage rate is normal if seizures controlled by age 12

Marriage rate is lower if uncontrolled seizures begin
before adolescence

Families are smaller than in general population

sensitive topic honestly, even when anonymous questionnaires are used. A woman whose husband is uninterested in sex or paternity can still have children, either by never using contraception and hoping that rare sexual encounters will result in pregnancy or by finding another sexual partner. If a man with an epileptic wife has a child with another woman, this child will not count in surveys of children produced by his marriage.

Married women with epilepsy seem to have fewer children than other married women simply because they do not become pregnant as often; their rates of miscarriage are no higher than those in the general population (14 percent). The seizure disorder itself does not seem to affect ovulatory cycles or cause hormonal problems that decrease fertility. Anticonvulsants have no apparent effects on the unfertilized eggs in a woman's ovaries, and the number of eggs released by women with epilepsy, whether on antiepileptic drugs or not, appears to be the same as that for women who do not have epilepsy.

Some women make a conscious decision not to reproduce. An epileptic woman in her late twenties told her new physician that both she and her husband had decided against having children for professional reasons. With a new regimen of antiepileptic drugs she became seizure-free within a month, after several years of poorly controlled complex partial seizures. After four months without seizures, she and her husband began asking about the dangers her drugs would pose to a fetus if she became pregnant. With the threat of seizures abating, the couple's views on having a family changed.

When seizures are well controlled, a parent with epilepsy can provide as much support, direction, and instruction for children as a parent without epilepsy. But the possibility that the disorder will cause problems in the future even though it is now under control inhibits some couples from becoming parents. The physician most familiar with the patient's seizure disorder should be able to estimate the future burdens likely to be imposed by the epilepsy. A parent with poorly controlled seizures cannot be relied upon to take full responsibility for a newborn infant, but the same person may be an excellent parent for a 4-year-old. A parent with frequent seizures should not be left to bathe the newborn alone but can play with and teach the older child. Obviously, the resources available to each couple and the roles each spouse is willing to play must be fully and objectively assessed when deciding whether or not to have children.

A recently married 28-year-old woman insisted that her career goals compelled her to avoid having children, but she contradicted herself when further questioned about her impressions of motherhood. She explained that her seizure disorder—generalized tonic-clonic seizures that recurred after years free of seizure activity—was of unknown cause and might be hereditary. She said her parents "had a nightmare with the epilepsy when I was a child. If it weren't for all the illness, they could have enjoyed themselves and had some money now." Though her father insisted that they had not suffered because of her epilepsy, she went on to discuss the special risks her child would face because she would have to take antiepileptic drugs throughout the pregnancy. Despite her avowed lack of interest in childbearing, she had accumulated a great deal of information on the birth defects associated with her anticonvulsants.

A person who wants to have a child but has an unwilling spouse has several options. If the marriage is of value to both spouses, professional counseling from either a marriage counselor or a sex therapist may be profitable. One option for a woman whose epileptic husband is impotent is artificial insemination. When the wife has epilepsy and does not want children, solutions available to the man who does not want to go outside his marriage are limited. If his wife is worried about pregnancy more than about raising a child, an impartial assessment by a physician of the risks involved for both the mother and the child may be helpful.

Potential parents who hesitate out of concern about inheritance of epilepsy should consult the physician most familiar with the patient's problem. The physician can give the couple a realistic estimate of the chances that a child will be affected. Occasionally the available information does not make it possible to say that a child will definitely have epilepsy or not, but the odds of having an unaffected child can usually be calculated.

Pregnancy

Women with epilepsy usually have uncomplicated pregnancies, normal deliveries, and healthy children. But it is also true that pregnancy presents special problems for the woman with epilepsy (Box 5.2). A woman who is on an antiepileptic drug must deal with changes in the way the medication is metabolized during the pregnancy, as well as with the effects the medication could have on the fetus. If she is on no medication, pregnancy may bring increased seizure activity. Even women who have never had seizures before may develop them during pregnancy. In that situation the question arises of whether to continue antiepileptic medication after the pregnancy has ended.

Effects of Pregnancy on Medication

Most anticonvulsants are metabolized more rapidly during pregnancy. This means that drug levels in the blood will fall as the pregnancy progresses and make the woman more vulnerable to seizures unless the dosage is increased. The rate at which the anticonvulsant level will fall is unpredictable; measuring the level every few weeks during the pregnancy is the best way to assess changes. An effective level can be maintained by simply increasing the dosage, but subtle factors, such as the binding of

---

**Box 5.2
Cautions with Pregnancy**

Metabolism of drugs changes

Seizure threshold may change

Anesthetic technique must be adjusted

Attention to sedation of the newborn

Attention to antiepileptics in breast milk

---

the drug to proteins in the blood, complicate the interpretation of drug levels. The additional dose required generally increases during the second and third trimesters of pregnancy, but the decision to change the dose of medication should be left to a physician familiar with the behavior of the drug and the pregnant woman's medical history. Increasing the amount of medication will not usually increase the side-effects. Most side-effects depend on what gets into the blood, not what goes into the stomach.

Any danger that medication may cause defects in the developing fetus is greatest during the first trimester of pregnancy, so there is no reason to allow the mother's level of anticonvulsant protection to fall during the second and third trimesters. Immediately after the end of the pregnancy, the dose of anticonvulsant required will decrease. To avoid an overdose at this point, the medication must be reduced, again with the rate of change dictated by changes in the level of anticonvulsant in the blood. Within a few months of delivery or termination of the pregnancy, the woman will usually require the same dose of anticonvulsants to control her seizures as she needed before she became pregnant.

Effects of Seizures on the Fetus

Good control of seizures is as important for the developing fetus as for the pregnant woman. Some women stop taking their anticonvulsant medication in anticipation of becoming pregnant or as soon as they realize they are pregnant. This places the fetus at risk of injury from seizures. Although the developing embryo will not develop seizures of its own simply because its mother is having seizures, it will have to deal with the profound metabolic changes that accompany some seizures. Generalized tonic-clonic (grand mal) seizures often start with abnormal or interrupted breathing. This causes a dramatic drop in the blood oxygen level, a sharp rise in blood carbon dioxide levels, and a coincidental rise in blood acidity. These changes, which may last minutes or hours, create an abnormal environment that may be harmful to the fetus. Additional damage to the fetus may occur if the woman injures herself during the seizure, a not uncommon occurrence with both generalized and partial seizures.

Effects of Pregnancy on Epilepsy

Pregnancy itself occasionally triggers seizure activity. When these seizures occur in association with high blood pressure, excessive swelling of the face and hands, and changes in kidney function, the woman is said to have eclampsia or toxemia of pregnancy. When the seizures occur without other apparent changes, they may be the first indication that the woman has epilepsy. Epilepsy routinely surfaces in vulnerable individuals under extraordinary stress. Pregnancy may not be an extraordinary physical stress for most women, but it does involve extraordinary hormonal changes, and these hormonal changes may uncover the seizure disorder.

Seizures that first occur during labor are more worrisome than those occurring earlier in the pregnancy, because they may be caused by bleeding from defects in the blood vessels of the mother's brain, brought on by the exertion and agitation of labor. Which women have the faulty vessels will not be apparent until the bleeding occurs.

For a woman with longstanding epilepsy, the exhaustion, pain, and lack of sleep associated with protracted labor may be stressful enough to induce a seizure. Minimizing the length of labor and the intensity of the pain has obvious advantages for the woman with a low seizure threshold, but this does not mean that a caesarian section is preferred for women with epilepsy. The indications for caesarian sections are the same for epileptic women as for other women. A caesarian section is more stressful for the woman than an uncomplicated vaginal delivery after a short period of labor. The simplest and least stressful approach to the delivery can only be decided by the woman's obstetrician. What happens during labor will affect the decision.

A seizure at any time during or shortly after pregnancy may be no more than the recurrence of a longstanding but unrecognized problem. Young women who develop seizures while pregnant may have no memory of seizures that they suffered in infancy. Because of the variety of possible causes of seizures during pregnancy, treatment is not a simple matter.

Any seizure not caused by an obvious metabolic problem should be treated with antiepileptic medication even if it occurs during the first trimester, the period during which the fetus is most sensitive to antiepileptic medications. If an obvious metabolic problem, such as a low level of calcium or sodium, is found, it should be corrected before anticonvulsant drugs are considered. Seizures caused by a correctable metabolic problem may be fully controlled without the use of anticonvulsant drugs. In all other situations an anticonvulsant should be given until the cause of the seizures can be established. Even if only one seizure has occurred and its cause is not apparent, antiepileptic medications should be prescribed. Seizures during pregnancy can never be viewed as benign incidents. They must be investigated and treated, regardless of when they occur in the pregnancy, but in both investigation and treatment the physician must consider risks to the fetus.

Both the mother and the physician should be reluctant to conduct extensive investigations during a pregnancy; those requiring radiation, such as a computed tomogram of the brain (CAT scan), or other tests that might damage the fetus should be delayed unless an induced abortion is planned. A spinal tap, in contrast, will not disturb the pregnancy and will reveal if bleeding has occurred into the spinal fluid. Ultrasound studies of the brain also pose no risk to the fetus and may provide evidence of abscesses, blood clots, or other large masses inside the head. A more thorough neurologic investigation with radiographic studies is appropriate after the pregnancy has ended. A woman who develops seizures during pregnancy may have a vascular malformation or a tumor that was not obvious until the stress of the pregnancy made the problem symptomatic.

Treatment of Seizures during Pregnancy

What medication should be used to suppress idiopathic seizures that first occur during pregnancy depends upon the type of seizure and the stage of pregnancy. If seizures appear during the first three months of pregnancy, the anticonvulsants most likely to cause birth defects should be avoided. This means that tri-methadione, phenytoin, primidone, and phenobarbital are in-advisable early in the pregnancy unless the woman was on these medications before she became pregnant. Whether phenytoin poses more of a risk to the developing fetus than primidone or phenobarbital is controversial. Any of these drugs should be avoided if possible. Other drugs occasionally used as antiepi-leptics, such as acetazolamide (Diamox), which do not consist-ently suppress seizures during pregnancy should also be avoided. Which medication is best for a particular woman depends on many factors, and both a neurologist and an obstetrician should be involved in the final decision. For many women, especially with complex partial seizures, carbamazepine is the drug of choice. Changes in the medication regimen early in a pregnancy have their own dangers and are not advisable.

If the seizures first occur during labor, an oral anticonvulsant may be impractical and an intravenous medication may pose unnecessary complications for the anesthesiologist. Intramus-cular phenobarbital may protect the patient from further seizure activity during the delivery without producing significant sed-ation of the mother or the newborn, though any antiepileptic given near the time of delivery must be considered a potential problem for the newborn as well as for the mother. If the dose of phenobarbital is relatively high, the physician must be pre-pared to deal with a sedated infant. However, there is no point in allowing the mother to face recurrent seizures to spare the child exposure to anticonvulsants. Both mother and newborn are best treated with effective anticonvulsant medication during labor, even if that means high intravenous doses of phenytoin, diazepam, or phenobarbital, and with close attention to blood pressure and breathing patterns in both.

Birth Defects

Most children born to women with epilepsy have no birth defects and never develop epilepsy. The incidence of birth defects in these children is greater than that in the general population, but it is still small. The incidence is only slightly increased for women with epilepsy who do not take anticonvulsants and do not have seizures during pregnancy, but it is five times greater than normal in women who use anticonvulsant drugs throughout pregnancy. The reason the rate is a bit higher even when no anticonvulsants are used is probably that some idiopathic seizure disorders are part of hereditary syndromes that can produce birth defects as well as epilepsy. The most common birth defects caused by antiepileptic drugs are cleft lip or palate, heart malformations, and hip dislocations. Cleft lip is 12 times as common as in the general population; heart anomalies are 18 times as common; and the relatively rare problem of congenital hip dislocation is 40 times as common.[2]

The risk faced varies with the drug taken. The highest rate of birth defects (12.7 percent) occurs in women who are taking multiple anticonvulsants and yet have seizures during pregnancy. The anticonvulsant most likely to cause fetal maldevelopment is trimethadione. Primidone, phenobarbital, and acetazolamide given during the first trimester also carry an increased risk. Serious facial, cardiac, or skeletal malformations appear in about one out of ten infants whose mothers take phenytoin during the first trimester, and the majority show temporarily slow growth and development. There is no way to predict how severely the infant will be affected by exposure to phenytoin; even twins may be affected differently. Carbamazepine and valproic acid have not been shown to increase the rate of birth defects, but the experience with valproic acid has been too limited to be conclusive. Diazepam (Valium) is not effective as an antiepileptic when taken orally, but it is effective against generalized seizures when given intravenously. Many women, whether they have epilepsy or not, take diazepam during pregnancy to deal with anxiety. The effects of this medication on the fetus are controversial, but current evidence suggests that it does not cause birth defects.

An unresolved question is what effect antiepileptic drug use by the father has on offspring. Most of the problems faced by the developing fetus are from exposure to antiepileptics while in the womb, but it is quite possible that sperm and eggs can be damaged before conception. If such damage occurs, it must be relatively rare for obvious defects to have eluded detection for so long.

Breastfeeding

Women who nurse their infants generally need not be concerned about the level of anticonvulsant medication in their milk. Some anticonvulsants, such as phenytoin, may be found in the milk in minute amounts, but they do not appear to cause problems for the developing infant. Of course, a woman should tell the physician prescribing any drug that she is breastfeeding.

The Inheritance of Epilepsy

Epilepsy usually appears in just one member of a family. It is easy to see why it is not properly considered a hereditary problem. The child of a man who develops epilepsy after a gunshot wound to the brain is at no greater risk of developing epilepsy than the child of a man shot through the lung is of developing shortness of breath. This is not to say that epilepsy never occurs in several members of a family. Some of the diseases that cause seizure disorders are inherited; this is why the likelihood of developing epilepsy increases if other members of an individual's family have epilepsy that is not caused by an injury or an infection in the nervous system.[3]

There are several patterns of inheritance for both normal and abnormal genetic traits. These generally are divided into dominant, recessive, and X-linked—designations indicating how the gene or genes responsible for the trait are transmitted from parents to children. Dominant traits can be inherited from either parent and will appear in half the offspring of an affected individual. Recessive traits appear only if a child inherits the gene from both parents. X-linked traits are carried on the X chromosome, which appears singly in men (who also have a Y chromosome) and as a pair in women. X-linked abnormalities usually appear only in men; in women the other normal X chromosome often compensates for any deficiencies in the abnormal X chromosome. Inheritance is more complicated than this simplified version: even when an abnormal trait is dominant, the likelihood that it will appear varies. The extent to which a defect is manifest, called its penetrance, may vary dramatically from one individual to another in the same family. Thus a father with tuberous sclerosis, a disorder with many possible nervous system complications, may pass on the gene for the disorder to his child, and yet the child may exhibit a much milder version of the trait than the father does.

Hereditary problems that may cause epilepsy include defects in brain formation, disorders of metabolism, and recurrent tumors. Occasionally an adult without epilepsy will have a hereditary neurologic disorder that can cause epilepsy in his or her offspring. The inherited defect need not be a nervous system malformation or a tumor but may be nothing more than an abnormality in electrical activity in the brain. Presumably such an abnormality results from a metabolic problem in the brain, but the chemical basis for it is simply not apparent with currently available tests.

The likelihood that any individual will develop epilepsy is 1 or 2 in 200. Considering all causes of epilepsy, the risk for a child with one epileptic parent is five times that of the general population, but that still places the risk at only 2 to 5 children out of 100. With some dominantly inherited seizure disorders, the risk that a child or a sibling of the affected person will have the disorder may be as high as 50 percent. Twins have an increased risk of both developing epilepsy if one does: this risk ranges from 5 to 20 percent for fraternal twins and from 40 to 90 percent for identical twins.

Considering the cause of the epilepsy, its type, and which parent has it, a child is at highest risk of developing epilepsy if the affected parent is the mother and she has generalized (petit mal or grand mal) seizures of unknown cause and with no aura (see Box 5.3). Regardless of which parent has the seizure disorder and what type of seizure the parent has, sons are slightly more likely to develop epilepsy than daughters. For the offspring of a parent with any one of several types of epilepsy, the incidence of seizures runs as high as 12 percent, but this disturbingly high figure includes children who have only one seizure in childhood and never develop a continuing epileptic problem. Unequivocal epilepsy will develop in 2.9 percent of the sons of women with all types of epilepsy, 2.3 percent of the daughters of women with epilepsy, 1.1 percent of the sons of men with epilepsy, and 0.6 percent of the daughters of men with epilepsy. Although the differences between these rates are small, they are statistically significant.

Why children of an epileptic mother are more likely to develop the problem than children of an epileptic father is unknown. Part of the statistical difference may be caused by mistaken identity: the wrong man is much more likely to be identified as a parent than the wrong woman. Another explanation is that birth complications play a part in the development of some seizure disorders, and women with epilepsy are more likely to have complicated pregnancies and deliveries than women without epilepsy.

Children who develop hereditary seizures unrelated to a metabolic problem follow a fairly predictable pattern. The seizures

---

Box 5.3
Factors Associated with an Increased
Risk of Inheriting Epilepsy

Mother has seizures

Offspring is male

Parent has idiopathic generalized seizures

Parent's seizures include no aura

Several members of the family have epilepsy

Metabolic disease known to cause epilepsy
occurs in relatives

usually appear between the ages of 5 and 19. The type of epilepsy is generally the same as that observed in the parent, but the age of onset for the child may be slightly earlier than that reported for the parent. A noteworthy exception to both of these rules occurs if the parent has simple partial (focal) epilepsy. Children of parents with simple partial epilepsies often develop generalized epilepsy, which usually surfaces by age 2 if it is going to develop at all.

Occasionally a child will be the first family member recognized to have epilepsy. Other relatives with "drop attacks," episodic confusion, blackouts, and temporary memory lapses will be diagnosed as suffering from epilepsy only after the child develops seizures. If a child has epilepsy, the likelihood that his parents have it may be as high as 14 percent; his siblings, 3 percent; his distant relatives, 2.8 percent. In some families a specific disorder causing seizures is not inherited but a general susceptibility to seizures of one type or another is inherited. A hereditary lack of resistance to viral infections of the brain, for example, may increase the likelihood that certain nerve cells in the brain will be damaged. The brain injury could cause epilepsy, and the epilepsy would appear more frequently in members of this family, even though the family members share a problem with immunity, rather than with the structure or function of the nervous system. This may explain the appearance of several different types of epilepsy in the same family. The most dramatic example of this is in the case of complex partial (psychomotor) seizures. Although most of the known causes of these seizures are not hereditary, 2.6 percent of the relatives of people who suffer from them will have some form of epilepsy.

Commonly Inherited Types of Seizures

Some types of epilepsy exhibit well-defined hereditary patterns. The classic form of petit mal is one of the most common hereditary types. True petit mal is transmitted in a dominant pattern, but individuals with a genetic predisposition to have this type of epilepsy do not necessarily have actual seizures. Adults who carry the gene or genes responsible for the disorder may exhibit the typical 3-per-second pattern of spikes and slow waves on their electroencephalograms even if they never have apparent seizures. A child will generally develop actual petit mal or absence seizures between the ages of 5 and 9 or not at all. Of those children whose electroencephalograms show the typical pattern, 25 percent will develop seizures. Thirty-five percent of the offspring of individuals with this electroencephalographic pattern will show the same pattern, at least during childhood, even if seizures never develop.[4]

Benign febrile seizures, which do occur more often in related individuals than in the general population, are not strictly speaking a form of epilepsy. Just as seizures will occur in some people who have low levels of calcium in their blood, seizures will occur in infants in some families when these children have high fevers. Benign febrile seizures invariably occur between 6 months and 4 years of age and only at the peak of a rapidly rising fever. The tendency to have these relatively benign and transient seizures appears to be transmitted in a dominant manner with variable penetrance.

A seizure disorder called Rolandic or benign focal epilepsy of childhood, which occurs in older children and resolves completely as the child matures, also seems to be dominantly inherited. Rolandic seizures may appear to be either focal or generalized, and attacks often occur during sleep. These seizures are easily controlled with anticonvulsants and stop by the end of adolescence.

Several different types of metabolic problems affecting the brain are inherited and cause epilepsy (see Chapter 10). In such cases the seizures may be the most obvious initial sign of the disease; this gives the false impression that the epilepsy, rather than the biochemical problem, is inherited. One such disorder is myoclonic photosensitive epilepsy, a dominantly inherited problem in which flashes of light precipitate seizures. The patient usually has a brief trance, often with small jerking movements of the limbs and trunk. On the electroencephalogram this may look very much like petit mal. Children may induce these seizures by waving their hands in front of their eyes or by watching a flickering television screen. This seizure disorder actually may be the initial sign of a metabolic disease, such as Lafora body disease, that causes central nervous system damage and produces a myoclonic epilepsy.

Hereditary Nervous System Diseases

Many hereditary diseases of the nervous system cause epilepsy as a symptom. The seizure disorder is rarely the only symptom of the hereditary disease, but it is quite often the initial or most prominent one.

DISORDERS APPARENT IN INFANCY. Most of the metabolic problems that cause seizures during infancy also cause mental retardation. Although the chemical bases for several of these disorders have been identified, treatment is available for very few.

Phenylketonuria (PKU), one of the most common causes of seizures and mental retardation in infants, is also one of the most treatable. The blood of a newborn can be checked for abnormal handling of the amino acid phenylalanine. If the tests indicate PKU, a diet low in phenylalanine may prevent significant retardation and epilepsy.

Even if a woman's phenylketonuria is well managed, so that she shows no sign of the disorder while on a careful diet, her children will be damaged by the disorder during their fetal development. The chemical abnormalities in the mother's blood, abnormalities that present no significant problems for the adult, may have a devastating effect on the developing fetus. These offspring invariably have intellectual problems and seizures because of brain damage induced by the mother's abnormal blood composition. This means that women with phenylketonuria should be advised against having children. The child of a woman with PKU is not likely to have PKU itself but is extremely likely to suffer severe nervous system damage.[5]

Another inherited disorder that can cause seizures is Tay-Sachs disease, a problem common in some groups of Ashkenazi Jews. As much as 3 percent of this population carries genes that will lead to a deficiency in the enzyme hexosaminidase A. Children who inherit this gene from both of their parents will develop seizures, progressive eye damage, and severe mental retardation. Tay-Sachs is a lethal disorder, and its victims rarely survive past 3 years of age. It can be detected in the sixteenth week of pregnancy by the procedure called amniocentesis, and the parents may choose to have an induced abortion before the defective fetus matures.

Less common, but equally lethal, metabolic disorders include several defects in metabolism of fatty materials (lipids). In Niemann-Pick, infantile Gaucher, and Krabbe disease, various materials accumulate abnormally in nerve cells and cause damage to the nervous system. In some diseases, this material has a waxy appearance after it is stained for pathologic study, and the disorders are called ceroid lipofuscinoses. All of these unusual metabolic disorders are recessively inherited.

There are several dominantly inherited problems that are relatively common and not invariably lethal. One of these is acute intermittent porphyria, an enzyme disorder that often causes problems with brain function.

Most of the X-linked diseases causing seizures are progressive disorders of the entire nervous system. In these disorders other symptoms are likely to overshadow the seizures, and the victims usually die in childhood. Treatment of seizures in these patients is frustrating because the progressive character of the diseases interferes with the development of an effective drug regimen.

TUBEROUS SCLEROSIS. Tuberous sclerosis is a hereditary disease that may cause little more than pale spots on the skin or may lead to profound mental retardation and epilepsy. It is a dominantly inherited disorder, and one child out of every 30,000 to 100,000 will develop the disease, but the severity of symptoms is remarkably variable and impossible to determine at birth. Common signs of this disease, other than seizures and mental retardation, include whitish spots on the skin, fibrous growths at the bases of the nails, and tumors in several different organs, including the brain, eye, kidney, and heart. Eighty-eight percent of people with the disease will have seizures, including all of those who also exhibit mental retardation. Sixty percent of the victims of tuberous sclerosis are retarded; and, if epilepsy develops before a child is 2 years old, that child will be retarded.

NEUROFIBROMATOSIS. Von Recklinghausen's neurofibromatosis, a hereditary disorder that affects the skeleton and skin as well as the nervous system, is dominantly inherited and appears in one out of 3,000 births. Twelve percent of the victims of this disease have seizure disorders, and many of these also have nervous system tumors, some of which are lethal. People with neurofibromatosis have lumps in the skin caused by benign tumors of the peripheral nerve lining cells and hyperpigmented spots, called café-au-lait spots, that extend over several centimeters. Although the condition is dominantly inherited, it has a variable penetrance. What type of seizures will develop with it is determined by what part of the brain is affected by abnormal structures or tumors. Many people with this disease remain free of seizures all their lives despite obvious tumors along nerves in the skin.

HUNTINGTON DISEASE. Huntington disease is a dominantly inherited disorder that usually causes abnormal movements and progressive intellectual deterioration. About 10 percent of patients with this disorder have seizures. There is also a "rigid" form of Huntington disease, which usually develops in children or adolescents, and which has a much higher incidence of seizures. These children experience rigidity, tremor, and diffuse slowing of movements similar to those of an elderly person with Parkinson disease. About 85 percent of children with this rigid form will have epilepsy. This is a slowly progressive disorder for which there is no treatment available.

Genetic Counseling

In a family with a clearly defined hereditary problem, it makes sense for couples to seek genetic counseling before they decide whether to have a child. The consequences of genetic counseling, however, have been disturbingly ironic. People who are told the risks of having a child with a hereditary disorder tend to have more children than similar people who are given no counseling. The parents of an affected child are inclined to suspect that any future child will be similarly affected. When they are told that the risk of having another child with the disorder is only one out of four or one out of two, they are more likely to have other children. Even if their second child also has, say, tuberous sclerosis, they assume that the probability of having a normal child increases if they simply keep trying. In fact, the risk that any particular child will be affected is exactly the same as that for previous children. If the risk of inheriting a nervous system disorder is fifty-fifty for the first child, it will be fifty-fifty for the tenth child, even if his nine siblings all have the disease. Genetic counselors must stress that inheritance is like coin-flipping: each flip of the coin is equally likely to turn up heads or tails, regardless of what turned up on previous tosses.

As more prenatal tests are developed to detect hereditary disorders that can cause epilepsy, more parents will be able to conceive, have the tests, and then decide whether to abort the fetus if it is abnormal. It would obviously be more desirable to avoid conceiving a defective fetus at all, but this type of genetic selection is still far from practical. Couples who are at high risk of having children with epilepsy should be given what information is available, including information on prenatal testing, and allowed to decide on a suitable course for themselves. If they decide to have no children or to adopt children, they should be directed to medical or social agencies that can help them realize these choices.

Chapter 6

Children with Epilepsy

Seizures are common in infancy, childhood, and adolescence. Some type of seizure activity occurs in as many as 8 out of every 1000 children. Occasionally the seizures disappear as the child matures, but in most cases epilepsy that appears in childhood will persist into adult life. About 80 percent of all people who have epilepsy are children or developed the problem when they were children. What family problems and conflicts will result from epilepsy in a child usually depends on the severity of the epilepsy. Well-controlled seizures may pose few real problems; poorly controlled seizures may become the focus of all family activities.[1]

With poor seizure control, parents often feel obliged to restrict the child's life and sometimes their own lives as well. The child may be preoccupied with fears that the seizures will be lethal or crippling. Even when seizures are fully controlled, family interactions that developed as a response to the earlier poorly controlled seizures may continue long after they are useful and appropriate. A mother's protectiveness may be necessary when close supervision is essential for seizure control, but if that same protectiveness persists after the seizures cease to be a problem, or even after the child becomes an adult, it can undermine the relationship between the mother and her child and make it difficult for the child to have a normal life.[2]

This same overprotectiveness sometimes forces a child with epilepsy into the role of being the permanently "sick" member of the family. The sick role evolves as the family's reaction to the threat of illness as much as to the reality of a chronic problem. Problems and fears that are appropriate only temporarily may be clung to indefinitely. The relationships that develop between the "sick" child, his or her parents, and his or her siblings may have disadvantages for each family member, but those relationships will still be difficult to alter.[3]

In fact, the outlook for families with children who have epilepsy is far from bleak. Children growing up with epilepsy can lead virtually normal lives. Seizure control is constantly evolving, with new medications and techniques regularly being introduced to minimize the effects of the disorder on both the child and the family. The results promise to make epilepsy a less and less disruptive force.

Causes of Epilepsy in Childhood

Children develop epilepsy for many of the same reasons as adults (see Chapter 10), but there are some noteworthy differences. Hereditary metabolic problems, with seizure disorders as an early symptom, are much more likely to appear in childhood than in adulthood (see Chapter 5), whereas brain tumors are more likely to cause seizures in adults than in children. Accidental poisoning (which can cause seizures) is a minor problem for adults but a major problem for children. Head injuries cause brain damage and seizure disorders at all ages, but children face different risks from head injuries at different stages in development of the skull and brain. There are also several problems that can occur only in infancy or childhood, such as infections and injuries suffered at birth. Children are not just small adults, and the causes, complications, and treatment of seizure disorders in infants and children must be viewed separately from those in adults.

Epilepsy in childhood may develop within hours of birth or late in adolescence. The age at which it appears is often related to the type of seizures or to their cause. Certain patterns of epilepsy, such as salaam attacks—brief episodes in which the child thrusts its arms forward as it drops its head—invariably appear in infancy. Others, such as myoclonic fits—seizures involving limb jerks that may knock the child to the ground without causing altered consciousness—are more typical of adolescence. If a metabolic problem is responsible for the seizures, the age of onset of seizures depends on the pace at which the metabolic disease disrupts the normal interaction of brain cells. Epilepsy may appear within the first few months of life in individuals with Tay-Sachs disease and not appear until adolescence in others with ceroid neuronal lipofuscinosis, even though both of these rare nervous system diseases involve the abnormal accumulation of materials in brain cells (see Chapter 5).

Congenital Disorders

Children are often born with the defect of the central nervous system that immediately or eventually causes epilepsy (see Box 6.1). This defect may be caused by an injury at birth, a hereditary metabolic problem, or a structural abnormality. When seizures developing in infancy or childhood can be traced to a discrete injury, the most common one is birth asphyxia, that is, inadequate oxygen to the brain during or just before delivery. Asphyxia is often presumed to be the cause of seizures in any child

---

**Box 6.1
Causes of Epilepsy in Newborns**

Birth asphyxia

Intrauterine infection

Metabolic disorders

Head injury

Congenital brain malformations

Intracranial hemorrhage

Drug withdrawal (with addict mother)

who had problems breathing at birth or who was delivered with the umbilical cord tightly bound around its neck. In fact, problems with breathing may be a sign of brain damage rather than the cause of it. Premature infants are especially vulnerable to bleeding in or about the brain, presumably because blood vessels in the head are fragile before the fetus has fully matured. This intracranial bleeding may be the unsuspected cause of both seizures and poor breathing in a premature newborn. Congenital metabolic disorders do not wait until after birth to cause their brain damage, and so some fetuses will have seizures and impaired brain development while still in the womb.[4]

In some instances, an infection acquired before or at birth causes brain damage that later produces slow intellectual development, limb weakness, poor coordination, or other neurologic defects. A variety of intrauterine infections, including toxoplasmosis and cytomegalovirus (CMV), may cause fetal brain damage that may result in epilepsy months or years later. Some infections are contracted during delivery, rather than while the fetus is developing in the uterus. For example, exposure to *Herpes simplex* in the birth canal may cause encephalitis that leaves the infant with a low seizure threshold. The risk of injury to the central nervous system is high enough that a caesarian section is often performed when this type of herpetic infection is evident in the birth canal.

Even when these other causes of perinatal damage are taken into account, birth asphyxia is the most common cause of brain damage at birth. Failure to provide the brain with adequate oxygen at birth produces an irreversible loss of nerve cells and changes in other elements of the brain. Epileptic activity develops from the increased irritability of the injured brain, and the extent of the damage determines what signs of nervous system injury besides the seizure disorder will appear as the child develops. Children with injuries caused by anoxia (insufficient oxygen) to the brain at birth are loosely grouped together under the term cerebral palsy. Epilepsy does not invariably develop with cerebral palsy, and when it does it may appear years after all other neurologic problems caused by the birth injury have stabilized.

Metabolic problems are often mistaken for cerebral palsy or, more precisely, for anoxic brain damage when the brain dysfunction is apparent within the first few weeks of life. If the metabolic disorder causes substantial damage to the gray matter of the brain, seizures often develop. The chemical or hormonal disturbance in this type of disease may be at a cellular or a glandular level. Tay-Sachs disease, for example, a hereditary disorder of a specific enzyme, causes intracellular failure to eliminate metabolic waste products. Other metabolic problems may result from impaired or inappropriate function of the thyroid, adrenal, pituitary, or other glands vital to normal growth and development.

Treatable metabolic disorders are exceedingly uncommon, but they are always worth looking for. One rare cause of seizures in newborns that can be treated is pyridoxine dependency. Infants with this disorder need high levels of pyridoxine, a B vitamin, in their diets to avoid mental retardation and seizures. More easily diagnosed metabolic problems include abnormal handling of calcium and magnesium. Chemical disorders of the blood are routinely tested for in the newborn period, and are usually easily corrected.[5]

In addition to hereditary errors of metabolism, such as Tay-Sachs disease and neuronal ceroid lipofuscinosis (see Chapter 5), seizures in childhood may also arise from developmental defects in the central nervous system. A child with a large port-wine spot on his face, for example, may have Sturge-Weber syndrome, a developmental abnormality that causes brain damage and vascular malformations with associated seizure disorders.

Head Injury

Brain damage from head injuries is very common in children (Box 6.2). Automobile accidents alone make head injuries a major public health problem, but added to this is the trauma sustained in falls, sporting injuries, and child abuse. The frontal and temporal lobes of the brain are especially vulnerable to contusion in the commonest form of head injury, in which the front of the head hits a hard object (Figure 6.1). In young infants, the bones of the skull are not fused and openings in the skull (fontanelles)

Box 6.2
Causes of Epilepsy in Children

"Cerebral palsy"

Head injury

Congenital malformations

Poisoning

Metabolic disorders

Nervous system infections

Brain tumors

Vascular malformations

---

are large enough to allow direct trauma to the brain. Efforts to mold the head by binding it tightly, a custom still practiced by several cultures around the world, can inadvertently cause trauma to the infant's poorly protected brain, but in most children the brain can survive such deformation without injury. Binding inflexible materials, such as wooden boards, over the fontanelles can cause injury to the brain, an injury that may not be manifest until years later when seizures appear. Brain injury may occur without any apparent skull fractures. In such cases, discharge of blood mixed with spinal fluid from the nose or ears of an infant may provide more unequivocal evidence of injury than a skull x-ray.

Child abuse can produce many long-term effects, one of which is seizure activity. That a child does not develop epilepsy within hours or days of a beating does not mean it will not subsequently have a seizure disorder. Children at special risk are those who lose consciousness with the beating and those who have evidence of skull fractures and intracranial blood clots. After a child who has been abused is protected from the abusive person, long-term observation for signs of epilepsy is appropriate.

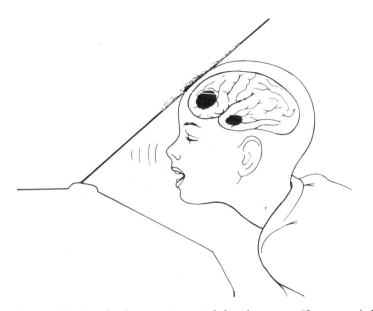

Figure 6.1 Cerebral contusions with head trauma. If a person's head strikes the windshield during an automobile accident, injury to the brain may occur. If there is structural damage, it is called a contusion and is often in the frontal or temporal lobes (shaded areas) of the brain. This bruised nerve tissue may be the site of origin for seizures in posttraumatic epilepsy.

In children as in adults, generalized tonic-clonic (grand mal) and complex partial (psychomotor) seizures are the most common types of seizures developing after head injuries. In most cases the character of the injury determines the type of seizure that develops, but in some cases a family history of seizures may lead to epilepsy after relatively minor head trauma. Children who are at no special risk of developing seizures may suffer major head trauma without ever having seizures. This simply means that a predisposition to develop epilepsy may be as important in some post-traumatic seizures as is the head injury itself. The treatment of post-traumatic seizures is determined by the type of seizure that develops. Changes in the pattern of epilepsy as the child matures require changes in the medications used to suppress the seizures.[6]

Febrile Seizures

Sometimes children with high fevers develop seizures, usually generalized convulsions entailing a loss of consciousness. Between birth and age 5, about 2 percent of all infants have febrile seizures and 1 percent have seizures unrelated to fevers. If the seizure occurs between 1 and 5 years of age, is associated with a fever, is nonfocal, lasts less than 15 minutes, and is not associated with a metabolic disorder or central nervous system infection, it is called a *simple febrile seizure*. This is distinguished from the *complex febrile seizure*, which lasts more than 15 minutes, has focal features, occurs before one year of age, or is associated with a family history of seizures. The distinction is important in determining treatment (Box 6.3). The simple febrile seizure does not call for antiepileptic therapy; the complex febrile seizure demands it.[7]

Box 6.3
Febrile Seizures

Simple	Complex
Characteristics	
Onset at 1–5 years old	Onset before 1 year of age
Generalized	Focal
Less than 15 minutes long	More than 15 minutes long
Obvious metabolic or infectious problem	Associated with history of seizures in family members
No apparent brain damage	Apparent neurologic trouble
Treatment	
Suppress fever	Anticonvulsants

Two out of three children with febrile seizures have simple febrile seizures. The likelihood that a child who has had a simple febrile seizure will ever have another febrile seizure is one in three. Of children exhibiting complex febrile seizures—seizures with any of the complicating factors listed—10 percent eventually will develop seizures without any associated fever. Of the children with simple febrile seizures, only 2.2 percent will develop convulsions not associated with fevers.

The reason children with simple febrile seizures are not treated with anticonvulsants when high fevers develop is that levels of anticonvulsant in the blood are achieved too slowly to make a difference when the child is acutely sick, unless the drugs are given intravenously each time a fever appears. The complication rate of intravenous anticonvulsant treatment is too high to justify its use with simple febrile seizures. But children with evidence of central nervous system damage should be started on anticonvulsant therapy after their first seizure, even if it is only a febrile seizure. Of children who have febrile seizures on more than three separate occasions, three out of five have a family history of febrile seizures and two out of three have abnormal brain waves. This simply indicates that the child and other affected family members have seizure thresholds low enough that relatively minor stimuli, such as high fevers, are enough to cause seizures. If one child in the family has febrile seizures, the likelihood that its sibling will also have febrile seizures is about 10–15 percent. If one identical twin has febrile seizures, the likelihood that the other twin will have them is several times greater than this. The more similar the genetic composition and intrauterine experience of two individuals, the more similar are their susceptibilities to epilepsy.

Occasionally a febrile seizure evolves into a string of seizures rather than just a single convulsion. This string of seizures may turn into an unrelenting and life-threatening condition called *status epilepticus*. The risk of this is greatest with a child's first febrile seizure. Therefore, any child experiencing his first febrile seizure should be admitted to a hospital for careful observation and evaluation. A child under 3 years of age may have meningitis. Signs of infection in and about the brain in infants can be extremely subtle. A lumbar puncture to check for infection in the cerebrospinal fluid may be the only way to determine whether an infection is responsible for an infant's seizure disorder. In children under 6 months of age, a life-threatening meningitis may show little more than fever and a seizure. In such cases the risks of lumbar puncture are far outweighed by the dangers of not detecting a meningitis early in its course.

If treatment of the seizure is warranted, phenobarbital is the drug of choice. Adverse reactions with this drug, which include irritability, hyperactivity, negativistic behavior, and rashes, occur in as many as half the children treated; but despite its disadvantages phenobarbital is preferred because of its relative safety. Alternative drugs such as sodium valproate can cause liver or pancreatic disease in rare patients. Pediatricians and pediatric neurologists do not use phenytoin for febrile seizures because of worries that this drug might slow growth and development in the very young child. Phenytoin does affect calcium metabolism and the availability of folic acid (a vitamin), but it is not obvious that it causes any more problems than phenobarbital. The long experience with and established safety of phenobarbital in the treatment of febrile seizures have made it the drug of choice, but this may change as other drugs with fewer side effects are developed. Problems with side effects necessitate stopping the drug in many cases, and as many as one in five parents stop giving the child the medication without consulting the physician.

Febrile seizures rarely occur in children after age 7. Children of 7 or older who develop seizures with high fevers should be investigated even more thoroughly than younger children. Common causes of seizures in these prepubertal children include tumors and central nervous system infections, both of which require early detection and treatment.

Poisoning

Poisoning is common in children because they so often swallow items they find lying around. The poisons likely to cause seizures are the same in children as in adults. In fact, children often take medications intended for adults; overdoses of aspirin and sleep medications are fairly common. Anticonvulsants are not necessary in such cases of poisoning unless recurrent seizures develop while the poison is being eliminated from the child's body. If a child takes an overdose of a barbiturate, seizures may not occur until the level of barbiturate in the blood begins to drop rapidly.

The one poison that particularly affects children is lead. They often ingest lead from soil, paint, plaster, and other materials that adults are not likely to swallow. Toxic levels of lead in the brain usually cause generalized tonic-clonic (grand mal) convulsions. Permanent brain damage from this poison may require long-term antiepileptic treatment.[8]

With every poison, the most important goal is to minimize the damage. Rapid clearance of the poison and close observation of the child during the time it takes to eliminate the poison are essential. If seizures are a prominent complication, anticonvulsants may be required for days or weeks after the poisoning. When children poison themselves with materials or medications they find around the house, their parents often feel terribly guilty. This guilt may make them watch the child too closely in the future. It is important for parents to avoid stifling the child with too many limitations and to take a rational approach to protecting the child from potential poisons. Repeated poisonings are common, but the child's curiosity is generally more at fault than the parents' carelessness.

Tumors

Brain tumors are a relatively rare cause of seizures in children. Some hereditary disorders, such as tuberous sclerosis (see Chapter 5), are associated with tumors in the brain during the first months of life; but even with these congenital problems, brain malformations rather than tumors are the usual explanation for seizures. Most childhood tumors occur at the base of the brain in the brainstem or the cerebellum, areas that do not cause seizure activity when damaged. These tumors may spread to the space overlying the brain and cause irritation that leads to seizures, but this is a later effect. What appears to be a tumor in a very young child should be investigated with a brain biopsy whenever that is feasible. Occasionally a local infection from tuberculosis, parasites, or other agents will masquerade as a mass in the brain. With a biopsy, the appropriate diagnosis and treatment can be reached.[9]

Seizure-Like Phenomena

Several phenomena that are easily confused with epilepsy occur in infants and children (Box 6.4). These behavioral abnormalities often involve choking or troubled breathing and may occur only during sleep. Vascular problems, such as migraine or abnormal reflexes, may be responsible for the worrisome behavior, but in many cases the disorder is caused by inadequate parental care. The best way to distinguish between these seizure-like phenomena and true seizures is to make electroencephalographic recordings during the abnormal phenomena. Brain waves may change during these episodes, but the patterns typical of true seizure activity, such as spikes, sharp waves, or bursts of slow waves (see Chapter 10), do not occur. When the electroencepha-

---

Box 6.4
Seizure-Like Phenomena

Esophageal reflux

Breathholding spells

Somnambulism (sleepwalking)

Somniloquy (sleeptalking)

Night terrors

Bruxism (toothgrinding)

Migraine

lographic recording is ambiguous, the setting in which the behavior occurs may be informative. If episodes happen only after an infant resists being fed, for example, the problem is more likely to be gastrointestinal or psychological than neurological.

Breathing Problems

At 6 to 8 weeks of age, some infants develop episodes of choking, during which they seem to have difficulty breathing. This develops without vomiting or any apparent regurgitation of food, and it is frequently associated with rigid extension or contortions of the arms and legs. The infant may arch its entire body and turn blue. This usually occurs in infants who have poor feeding patterns and whose parents leave them to cry for long periods to get attention. Although no epileptic activity is occurring, the child is usually regurgitating food into its esophagus. Holding the child while it is fed and for some time afterward is often all that is required to eliminate this disturbing behavior. Without this change in parent-child contact, the regurgitation may persist for months.

Older infants and children may have spells of holding their breath. These spells occur in as much as 5 percent of the general population, and one out of four children with this behavior has another family member with a history of similar spells. These spells generally appear between 6 months and 4 years of age. The child stops breathing for several seconds or minutes and may turn pale or blue. In some infants the problem is a transiently overactive vascular (vagal) reflex that causes a marked slowing of the heart rate. In most, it is a behavioral abnormality associated with protracted anger and frustration. If an overactive vagal reflex is responsible, the behavior will abate as the child matures. If the child is holding his breath in reaction to excessive frustration, other behaviorial abnormalities are likely to appear as he gets older. Parents can minimize such breathholding spells and avoid future behavioral problems by spending more time interacting with the child. Parents should provide no rewards for breathholding, but should give consistent incentives for more constructive behavior.

Sleep-Related Disorders

Sleepwalking, sleeptalking, and night terrors are not caused by seizure activity, but features of each of these nocturnal phenomena resemble seizure activity enough to confuse physicians as well as parents. The parents are especially likely to suspect epilepsy if another family member has seizures. Seizures do sometimes occur during sleep and can induce the child to walk, talk, or appear acutely frightened; but seizure activity usually also appears when a child is awake and produces other signs of abnormal brain activity, such as generalized convulsions, postictal confusion, and premonitory auras. With both seizure activity and sleep phenomena, the child does not recall the abnormal behavior when fully awake. The confusion, irritability, and combativeness exhibited by children during these episodes support the notion that abnormal brain activity akin to epilepsy is responsible, but an electroencephalogram will establish that epilepsy is not involved.

Grinding of teeth (bruxism) sometimes arouses concern, but it is so common in the general population that it rarely warrants any investigation. Bedwetting (enuresis), usually a benign sleep phenomenon in very young children, may also be a sign of seizure activity in sleep. Unlike sleepwalking, sleeptalking, and night terrors, bedwetting is usually dismissed by parents as an embarrassing incident rather than considered a worrisome sign. This dismissal may be a mistake, especially if the child is entering puberty or late adolescence at the time of the bedwetting.[10]

Migraine

Migraine headaches in children can cause confused states, memory disturbances, and disorientation, but the pattern of pain and a family history of migraine usually simplify the identification of this problem. Migraine pain is usually on one side of the head and may be centered about or over one eye or temple. The pain lasts minutes to hours and is sometimes associated with nausea and vomiting. Visual changes often warn of an impending migraine.

Basilar artery migraine can be more difficult to diagnose because it involves blood vessels supplying the base of the brain. Symptoms that develop with basilar artery migraine include vertigo, gait disorders, double vision, and vomiting. This type of migraine is especially common in adolescents and young adults. Complicating its recognition as migraine rather than epilepsy is the common finding of spikes in the occipital (posterior) part of the head on the electroencephalogram. In many cases, a trial of medication to suppress the migraine headache will help sort out the patients with a vascular disorder from those with a seizure disorder.

Learning and Behavior Problems

Most children who have epilepsy without any other nervous system disease do as well in school as their peers and have no obvious personality disorders. But there are exceptions. Problems with learning ability and behavior most commonly appear when there are other neurologic signs in addition to seizures, such as limb weakness or impaired coordination. Overall, children with epilepsy have more behavioral and learning disorders than either healthy children or children with other chronic nonneurologic disorders, such as lung or heart disease. Intermittent disturbance of brain activity certainly plays a role, but parental attitudes and expectations can profoundly influence the child's social and academic performance. Expecting the child to be unable to perform at a level appropriate for his age and intelligence seems to ensure that he will not.[11]

Behavioral problems occur in many different kinds of epilepsy and involve many different kinds of behavior. One of the more obvious problems is violent or destructive actions. The type of epilepsy the child has appears to influence whether or not this destructiveness will develop. Children with complex partial (psychomotor) and generalized tonic-clonic (grand mal) epilepsy exhibit slightly more violent behavior than children with more focal seizure disorders. Both boys and girls are more likely to be violent if they have generalized seizures that first develop after 14 to 18 years of age. Several types of behavior disorders, not necessarily including violent or destructive actions, are especially likely in boys with complex partial seizures. These may involve difficulty in socializing with other children, dealing with failure, participating in family activities, and meeting other common demands of childhood. Destructive behavior is also common in children with the rare generalized nonconvulsive epilepsy called akinetic epilepsy. Violent behavior is not common in children with myoclonic seizures. With all types of epilepsy and all types of abnormal behavior considered together, 25 percent of the children with seizure disorders develop psychosocial problems severe enough to justify or require professional attention.[12]

Problems in School

Learning is sometimes a problem for children with epilepsy. Learning disorders are often exaggerated because of the common misconception that epilepsy and mental retardation are related. For children without mental retardation, whether a learning disability occurs is influenced by the age at which the epilepsy first appears: the later epilepsy develops, the lower the child's risk of learning problems. This is probably because disorders that cause both diffuse brain damage and epilepsy are more likely before 1 year of age than at other ages. Whatever the reason, children at ages 9 to 15 with generalized convulsive seizure disorders are significantly less impaired on tests of neuropsychological performance if their seizures began when they were between 8 and 14 than if they began before age 5. Tasks that require coordination, protracted attention and concentration, complex problem solving, or good memory function are especially difficult for children with very early (0–5) and relatively late (14–18) age of onset of seizures.

Children with idiopathic epilepsy, as a group, are much less likely to show impaired intellectual function than are children with symptomatic epilepsy. This is part of the reason for the poorer performance of children who develop epilepsy late in adolescence. These children are less likely to have idiopathic seizures than children whose epilepsy develops at about the time of puberty, and they often have seizures caused by infections and trauma.[13]

The reason that children whose epilepsy develops before age 5 also do more poorly as a group is probably that that group includes children impaired by birth asphyxia, intrauterine infections, brain malformations, and other causes of congenital brain damage. Such brain-damaged children usually develop seizures before their first birthday. The poorer intellectual performance of children whose seizures begin before age 5 is *not* caused by an adverse effect on the brain of either the seizures themselves or the anticonvulsants used to suppress the seizures.

Regardless of his or her intellectual abilities, the child with epilepsy is unavoidably treated differently in school from other children. Even the most understanding teachers carry their own fears and misconceptions of this disorder. The teacher is often worried about inadvertently causing a seizure. Many parents have grossly inaccurate beliefs about epilepsy that they pass on to the teacher. A mother who has seen her child turn blue during a generalized convulsion may confide in the teacher that the last seizure nearly killed the child. The epilepsy takes on life-threatening dimensions, and all but the most enlightened teachers will be terrified by the prospect of a seizure occurring in the classroom. The parents' excessive protectiveness is transferred to the classroom, and special treatment may isolate the child from classmates.

If the teacher does not know the child has a seizure disorder, the impact of a seizure that occurs at school will be even greater. Children with generalized absence (petit mal) epilepsy are often accused of daydreaming, since absence attacks are difficult to differentiate from inattentiveness. The child may be disciplined for laziness or disobedience. Teachers unfamiliar with seizure disorders may mistake a generalized convulsion for a fainting spell or a psychomotor attack for temporary insanity. Even if the teacher can be convinced that the harrowing experience was caused by a relatively benign neurological disorder, the teacher's understandable reluctance to be burdened by the problem will interfere with the child's experience at school.

Children with epilepsy are commonly reported by their teachers to be solitary, irritable, uninterested, and unpopular. Much of this behavior may result from the child's recognition that he or she is different from other children, and from the fact that in school the child does not hold the pivotal role held at home, even if the teachers are protective. These children often lag months or years behind their age group in school. Their teachers ascribe this slow advancement to the effects of medication and to parental attitudes. In fact the problems are often exacerbated by the attitudes of the teachers themselves, who may share the common misconception that epilepsy equals mental retardation and so may reduce their expectations of the child.

The relatively poor adjustment and achievement in school of children with epilepsy are usually unrelated to any nervous system problem; intelligence tests indicate that they should perform much better than they do. At least part of this underachievement grows out of parents' expectations that the child with epilepsy will do less well in social activities, sports, and scholastic achievement than the child without epilepsy. These expectations are imposed upon the child in a fairly obvious way. Parents seek to excuse the child from sports and other strenuous activities, for example, a maneuver that not only announces the child's problem to classmates and reinforces his sense of being different, but also encourages his withdrawal and isolation.

The child's teachers would be helped greatly by an unambiguous statement from the physician of what the child can and cannot do. The physician should give this information directly to the teachers rather than sending it through the parents. If the child is at risk of having seizures, the teacher must be told what to expect and what to do. Despite oppressive parental fears, the real dangers faced by the child who has a seizure in school are minimal. The child should not be kept out of sports and other activities, unless his or her particular type of epilepsy poses special risks.

Parents' Limited Expectations

Ideally, every parent with an epileptic child should have an accurate view of what the child's potential is and should help the child to achieve that potential, both at school and at home. Unfortunately, many parents fall short of this ideal. Parents often impose excessive limits on the child with epilepsy, perhaps as an overreaction to their inability to control the child's seizures. Or the overprotectiveness may be an attempt to compensate for injury they imagine they have inflicted on the child. Many parents have a nagging conviction that the child would be fine if they had acted differently. The guilt may take on a religious quality: the parents may see themselves as being punished for a religious transgression, and so they may feel especially responsible for the affliction visited upon their innocent child.[14]

Of course, many families who limit the goals they set for their children do so out of neglect rather than overresponsibility. The family may have assigned the child the role of cripple and may be reluctant to release the child from that role. Many parents admit that they see their child with epilepsy as a pitiful, unfortunate person who should not be expected to achieve anything. Unfortunately, the child with epilepsy, like any child, incorporates his parents' opinions about himself. If the parents believe that the child cannot achieve anything substantial, the child soon believes it too. Many children with epilepsy have inappropriately low aspirations and become very dependent in interpersonal relationships.

Children with epilepsy often have trouble developing relationships with other children. They tend to be isolated from their peers but inordinately dependent upon their mothers. This failure to socialize develops partly because of parental restrictions. The parents lack confidence that the child can manage outside the family if a seizure occurs, and a seizure can occur at any time. The child adopts this parental attitude and clings to the family.

To allow the child to grow into a normal, capable adult, the parents must be willing to involve the child with the world outside the family. Recreational camps, extramural school activities, and other well-structured settings in which the child can mix with other children are very beneficial. The parents should encourage the child to participate in such activities. Involvement with people outside the immediate family will make the child more flexible and resourceful even if the parents have trouble shedding their own limited expectations.

Behavioral Effects of Antiepileptic Drugs

Treatment of epilepsy is no more complicated and no less successful in children than it is in adults, but some adverse reactions that develop in children on antiepileptic drugs rarely appear in adults. Some of the difficulty with learning and behavior observed in children with epilepsy may be an effect of their anticonvulsant medication. Phenobarbital is being used less each year as alternative anticonvulsants are introduced (see Chapter 11), but many physicians still use it to treat generalized seizures in childhood. One of its side-effects is hyperactivity. Although phenobarbital is a sedative in adults, it may arouse children to excessive and sometimes destructive behavior. Children taking phenobarbital are often inattentive, irritable, aggressive, and tearful. Primidone, a drug popular in the treatment of complex partial seizures, can have many of the same side-effects as phenobarbital. Hyperactivity may be so disruptive to the child and his family that other anticonvulsants must be tried until a more suitable drug is found.[15]

Generalized absence (petit mal) seizures are usually treated with ethosuximide, which occasionally causes irritability directly or by interfering with sleep. Children on ethosuximide have a special susceptibility to night terrors, frightening images that occur during sleep and often awaken the child. Myoclonic and other types of epilepsy that do not respond to conventional anticonvulsants are often treated with clonazepam, which can cause withdrawn behavior, mood swings, and auditory hallucinations.

Sometimes behavioral problems such as hyperactivity appear but are unrelated to either the medication or the seizure activity itself. For many of these children, temper tantrums, poor tolerance of frustration, and hyperactivity improve with age, rather than with any specific treatment. Children with behavioral problems that do not respond to changes in medication and that do not improve with age usually have obvious structural damage to the brain. In fact, structural brain damage and intellectual impairment resulting from undiscovered brain damage are more often responsible for hyperactivity and destructiveness in children than is any social factor.

Conflicts within the Family

Epilepsy in a child unavoidably disturbs the normal relationships in the family. This disturbance grows out of the child's self-image as well as the way the rest of the family sees the child. Rather than developing a sense of competence, the child with epilepsy early on experiences an inability to control the forces acting on him or her. In many families, fear and insecurity are magnified in the exchange between child and parents. Both the child and the parents are uncomfortably aware of their inability to control the epilepsy. Parents may have excessive concern for the child's well-being, may strenuously deny his problem, or simply may reject him because of his chronic disorder. Often the parents' feelings toward the child involve an element of shame. This embarrassment over having a chronically ill child is rarely overt, but it is apparent to the child.[16]

Parents rarely seek authoritative information on seizure disorders. One-third of parents with children with epilepsy never discuss the disorder with the child with any frankness. The parents are frightened by the seizures and often have no idea of what to do when one occurs even if they have discussed them with a physician. More than half never read anything about epilepsy, but they do gather considerable hearsay from friends and relatives. This fosters misconceptions that may be damaging to the child.

Because they do not understand the causes and consequences of their child's epilepsy, many parents are most comfortable raising the child according to arbitrary and highly restrictive guidelines. The more inflexible the parents are, the more of a problem the epilepsy is likely to be. Even seizure control is related to the parents' attitudes. Children with autocratic parents have poorer seizure control on antiepileptic drugs than do children with less restrictive parents. Children do best, at least in terms of seizure control, in families that allow them a normal level of independence and discipline.

Manipulation of Parents by Children

Parents usually treat children with epilepsy the way they would any sick child. The problem with this approach is that most illnesses are transient, whereas epilepsy continues for years or a lifetime. Unless the parents are unusually well-informed, they are likely to worry that they will inadvertently make the epilepsy worse. Even if they know that their every action and remark will not significantly affect the disorder, each severe attack will stir up the notion that the child might have fared better if they had behaved differently.[17]

Children quickly realize that parental fears and guilt are easily played upon. Any attempts to discipline the child can be subverted by the threat that such treatment will cause a seizure. This manipulation of the parents aggravates an already difficult family situation and evokes much resentment, a resentment that is often not recognized by the individuals experiencing it.

CAPITALIZING ON PARENTAL GUILT. A child with severely disabling seizures imposes restrictions on the family that may make the child a virtual tyrant over the family. All family activities may be fashioned around the child's limitations. Parents who are angry at these limitations may feel very guilty because of this anger.

In their guilt, the parents may give in to the epileptic child's every whim, always believing they only want to do what is best for the child. The child who is frightened of traveling may become ill whenever a trip is planned. The parents may worry about what effect travel actually has on the child, but they cannot help resenting the limitations placed on them by the neurologic condition. To avoid conflict, the parents may check with the child before making plans. The child, frustrated by being unable to control the epilepsy, finds that he has considerable control over family activities. He may even pretend to have seizures at various times as a way of gaining control over circumstances in his own life (see Chapter 10).

A balance must be struck between the needs of the patient and the needs of the entire family. To minimize the likelihood of a power struggle with the patient, the parents must be consistent and fair. The child must be shown that intimidation will not work and that illness is not beneficial. When a trip is planned, it should be carried out. If he seems to be unable to participate in a family activity, then alternative arrangements should be made for the care of the child; the family should not give up the activity. The entire family should not be governed by the whim or illness of the epileptic child, and the child should be able to rely upon the parents' judgment when an activity is planned.

SELF-INDUCED SEIZURES. One young woman whose psychomotor seizures were not diagnosed until she was well over 20 years old recalled amusing herself as a child by rotating a mayonnaise jar in the refrigerator as fast as she could. The rotating pattern would bring on visual hallucinations, including a hula dancer, that she found fascinating. These were sensory seizures that she induced in herself by moving the jar, and she later developed complex partial seizures with visual hallucinations as part of the aura. She did not tell her parents about these hallucinations and never considered tham at all peculiar until questioned about the different types of hallucinations she developed as an adult. Many children discover that they can trigger seizures with certain stimuli, and usually at about the same time they discover the power they can exert in the family by having seizures.

A child who can bring on his own seizures is in a powerful bargaining position in the family. He has the option of simply becoming sick if the adults do not do what he wants. He can make seizures occur at very inopportune times if he chooses. This behavior will bring the most unbending parent to compromise. The main disadvantage of this maneuver is that the child in the sick role is excluded from many activities that he might enjoy.

To minimize this type of activity, it is important to be sure the child is not rewarded for it. A seizure, real or otherwise, should not consume all of a parent's energies. The spouse and the other children have equally legitimate claims on the parent's attention and affection, and they should not be neglected. Ascribing too much importance to seizures and giving them too much attention encourages the child to exploit them.

Parental Control of the Patient's Life

Parents often react to their inability to control the seizures by extending their influence and protection over inappropriate areas of the child's life. One out of three parents of children with epilepsy believes that the children require constant supervision, even after the seizures have been completely controlled for months or years. Parents encourage passivity in these children and discourage self-reliance and initiative. Eating habits, friendships, travel patterns, and play may all be regulated with an inappropriate and unproductive strictness. The struggle to control the child is disguised as a wish to protect him. All excitement is banned because of the risk of seizures. No opportunities to fail are allowed, even if that failure will be instructive. Any activity that makes the parent nervous is forbidden because "it may cause fits." Exaggerating their legitimate concern that a seizure may occur in a dangerous situation, the parents may constantly monitor and restrict the child's activities.[18]

PARENTAL FEARS AND DENIAL. Parents are often frightened by their lack of control over seizure activity. At its worst they may be constantly terrified that the child will die during a seizure while they stand by helplessly. How they react to this impotence varies. Some simply deny that their child has any problem at all and insist that the child could be like any other children if he or she wanted to.

Denial of the problem is less common than overattention to it. When parents do ignore all the precautions that are appropriate for a child with seizures, they may claim they are following the physician's instructions. If the physician uses euphemisms to refer to the epilepsy, the parents may take this lack of frankness as evidence that the problem is not epilepsy or that epilepsy is too terrible to discuss forthrightly. Some parents avoid telling the child what his problem is and pretend that the medication is a vitamin or a pill for a less serious disorder. Whatever attitude the family members take early on is likely to harden as the condition continues.

LONG-TERM EFFECTS OF PARENTAL INTERFERENCE. Even when parents' efforts to limit the child's activities are successful, they are usually only temporarily so. Restricting the child's autonomy backfires in most cases because the child eventually either rebels against all rules or becomes passive and dependent upon the restrictive parents. In early childhood the most common reaction is passivity and withdrawal. The child interacts with parents and siblings as little as possible and accepts parental decisions without resistance. This response to excessive restriction is often misconstrued by the parents as an effect of the epilepsy itself or of the medication. It is important to recognize the behavior for what it is, if only to minimize problems when the child becomes more independent. Unfortunately, a well-established pattern of dependence upon their parents leaves many children ill-prepared to manage the epilepsy and to take responsibility for other aspects of their lives when they become adults.

In some families the child with epilepsy fills a real need, that of keeping the parents together. The parents may have little holding them together besides the child's dependence upon them; and if one of them wants the marriage to continue, the child's dependence may become an indispensable element in the family. Any attempts by the child to be independent will undermine the relationship between the parents. Thus the parents treat the child as helpless regardless of his or her real abilities and needs. The couple can also avoid dealing with their own conflicts by focusing their resentment and frustration on the child's chronic problem. The family becomes centered upon the child simply to survive.

Even when the person with seizures is not exploited to stabilize the family, the epilepsy itself lends a distinctive character to the way the family functions. Families with an epileptic child are more disciplined than other families. This is true even when the child has been seizure-free for more than six months. Problems are solved in an efficient, albeit tyrannical, manner. The hierarchy is much more evident and rigid in these families than in families without epileptic children, and this hierarchy is not quickly disassembled after its organizing influence is no longer needed. The mother assumes an inordinately dominant position if she is primarily responsible for the child. Apparently this rigid family structure not only serves the child's needs to be protected and supervised but also protects the family from the disruptive effects of the disorder.

PROTECTION FROM FAILURE. This rigid pattern of family interactions can limit the child's ability to cope outside the family. By sheltering the child from failure, the parents keep him from becoming independent. The most routine tasks, such as preparing food, shopping, and choosing clothing, may be taken over by the parents in the unspoken belief that the child could not do them without failing. The suspicion that the child is not competent to take on routine tasks may be accurate in some cases, but parents who do not give the child a chance to be responsible for such activities ensure that he will never become competent.

CONSTRUCTIVE MEASURES. Dealing with children whose epilepsy is poorly controlled is certainly not simple, but there are some techniques that can minimize the difficulties. The family must know precisely what the child's problem is. Fantasies about epilepsy, which occur in even the most sophisticated families, are counterproductive. All fantasies must be explored and discarded. Blaming the epilepsy on some member of the family is especially disruptive. Accusations of blame are a poorly disguised attempt by the family members making the accusations to dissociate themselves from the problem.

The family should focus on what the child *can* do. Abilities, rather than disabilities, should be emphasized. As the child matures, he or she should be encouraged to be responsible for taking medication and observing reasonable precautions. The child should be allowed to deal directly with physicians. Career goals should be fostered with as little reference to the seizure disorder as possible. A child hoping to be a jet pilot should obviously be informed of the impossibility of this line of work for a person with epilepsy, but very few fields are so inflexible. Problems that develop because of the epilepsy should be discussed, but not obsessively, and honesty inside and outside the family should be encouraged. The child has nothing to be embarrassed about or ashamed of and should be treated accordingly by the parents.

The Adolescent with Epilepsy

Epilepsy presents several new problems in adolescence. The crucial issues at this time of life are independence, identity, and conformity, all of which are complicated by epilepsy and its treatment. In the United States, part of the independence that comes with adolescence is getting a driver's license. Many adolescents deny that they have epilepsy if admitting it is likely to prevent them from driving. Part of denying the epilepsy is not taking medication, a practice the adolescent usually identifies with overbearing parents anyway. Peers are likely to question any drug taking and treat someone they know to have epilepsy as different. Medication and visits to the physician become a focus for issues of control between adolescents and their parents. Refusal to take medication is especially common when control is incomplete but the seizures that persist are not totally disabling. The apparent ineffectiveness of the medication makes the adolescent more inclined to resent attempts to regulate his life, a life that is disrupted by the threat of seizures. Children with relatively minor seizure disorders may have worse social adjustment than those with severe epilepsy because they feel more annoyed than burdened by the seizures and more burdened than helped by the anticonvulsants. They see themselves repeatedly frustrated in trying to have the lifestyle of their peers, a lifestyle independent of medication and of many restrictions on their activities. Adolescents who have more frequent or more severe seizures usually are more cooperative in following medication recommendations and activity restrictions.[19]

A high school student who had concealed her generalized seizures from her friends for years was determined to try out for the swimming team even though she had never been an avid swimmer, because all her friends were on the team. Her mother forbade her to go swimming, but she ignored this restriction even though she knew she faced a real danger. She told her mother that she knew what she was doing, and that if she was going to die, she was at least going to die happy. She did not drown, and her seizure disorder certainly did not make swimming impossible. But her main reason for joining the team was to demonstrate to her friends that she needed to observe no precautions. This recklessness had developed in opposition to her family's excessive cautiousness.

ABUSE OF ANTICONVULSANTS. In a culture prone to drug abuse, the epileptic adolescent's unlimited access to controlled drugs can provide an easy route to popularity. The sale or free distribution of barbiturates by adolescents with epilepsy is enough of a problem in some cities to require highly regulated access to these medications. Some of these adolescents themselves abuse the drugs; after years of resisting parental pressure to take the medication, they experiment with excessive doses of anticonvulsants. Regular checking of serum blood levels will help detect much of this abuse, but the best approach is simply to switch to anticonvulsants without any resale value or well-recognized potential for abuse, such as phenytoin, carbamazepine, or valproic acid.

ABUSE OF ALCOHOL AND OTHER DRUGS. Alcohol and other drugs used for recreation alter the metabolism of anticonvulsant drugs. Adolescents exhibit as little judgment in using alcohol, barbiturates, and other intoxicants as adults do. Excessive alcohol intake makes an individual more vulnerable to seizure activity. The seizures occur when the level of alcohol or barbiturate in the blood falls. If the adolescent has concealed the drug abuse, the parents may take him to the doctor in extreme anxiety over the renewal of epileptic activity. Abuse of drugs of any kind is more severe in families where the adults have their own addictions. A child who is ordered not to drink alcohol by a parent who drinks every day is likely to ignore the instruction. Parents who are dependent upon sedatives or other types of relaxants are poor models for children who must be careful in their use of drugs.

Parental Inflexibility as the Child Matures

Emily's mother insisted that if Emily would only do what her parents repeatedly told her to do she would not have recurrent seizures. The mother blamed recent seizures on Emily's erratic sleeping schedule, poor diet, excessive socializing, and rowdy friends. With obvious sincerity, the concerned mother told Emily's physician, "I've told her many times that I disapprove of her behavior." The daughter was 34 years old, married, with children of her own, but her mother still treated her the same way she had when Emily developed seizures at 5 years of age. Emily resented her mother's prying and described her mother as an ever critical, disruptive force that she could not escape. The mother blamed the seizure activity on whatever behavior she disapproved of and took her complaints to her son-in-law when her daughter refused to listen to her.

This is an example of a common problem: many parents treat their epileptic child in the same way for decades. Finding a way to cope with the seizure disorder is so difficult for most parents that they seem unable to adjust their strategies as the child gets older. Such inflexibility leads to a progressive alienation of the person with epilepsy from the family. This pattern also contributes to the isolation felt by many adults with epilepsy.

Prognosis

Even before anticonvulsants were discovered, many seizure disorders disappeared within months or years of their appearance. This is still true. Of the people who consult a doctor within a year of the appearance of episodes that are thought to be seizures, as many as 85 percent have spontaneous remission of their disorder. This drops to 50 percent for people who are not seen by a physician until the episodes have persisted for more than a year, but this simply means that if the problem is epilepsy and the epilepsy is going to disappear on its own it will often do it within a year of its appearance.

Different types of seizures exhibit different tendencies to remit. Generalized absence (petit mal) seizures often abate late in adolescence and leave the patient with no signs of brain damage. Infantile spasms, in contrast, usually lead to devastating neurologic problems in the children who survive with this type of seizure disorder. Anticonvulsants have not substantially affected the remission rates of different types of epilepsy. What they have affected is the harm done by the seizure disorders. Aside from the obvious social toll to the individual and the family, an active seizure disorder poses real medical risks. Frequent seizures in children may even contribute to a deterioration in their intellectual abilities, not necessarily because of brain damage but simply because of the restraints on intellectual development imposed by frequent seizures. The risk of premature death is also increased, because children with seizures face a higher risk of accidents than children without them.[20]

Treating a First Seizure

Aside from the controversy surrounding the treatment of febrile seizures, there are other seizure disorders in which real questions exist about whether a single seizure justifies treatment. In children many seizure disorders occur repeatedly before they are even suspected. The initial absence attack or myoclonic seizure usually goes unnoticed or is ascribed to tiredness. These seizures demand treatment when they are finally recognized. Seizures that occur only when the child is asleep also require investigation and treatment. Nocturnal seizures are just as serious as those which occur when the child is awake and active. More controversial is what to do for a child who has his first grand mal, focal sensory, focal motor, or psychomotor seizure.

The risk of subsequent seizures can be estimated according to the cause of the seizure, the incidence of epilepsy in the family, and the electroencephalographic pattern observed after the child has recovered from the seizure, but this estimate is not a guarantee that seizures will or will not recur.[21]

The child's age at the initial seizure, the type of seizure observed, and any neurologic abnormalities that might be found on first examining the child do not indicate the risk of recurrence of the seizure. Even if the first seizure episode is status epilepticus, later seizures may not develop once that first episode has passed. Of individuals who have an idiopathic seizure and epileptic siblings, 35 percent have another seizure within four months. Abnormal brain wave patterns may persist for years without any further actual seizures, but a generalized spike and slow wave pattern on the electroencephalogram when a patient has fully recovered from his first seizure does indicate a high likelihood of recurrent seizures. Half of the patients with this electroencephalographic abnormality will have another seizure within 18 months. If spikes appear over the central temporal area, the risk of recurrent seizures may be even greater. When the electroencephalogram is normal or has nonspecific abnormalities, the likelihood that an idiopathic seizure will be followed by a second seizure within two years is only 14 percent.

If the initial seizure follows a significant head injury, the risk of a second seizure within 20 months is 46 percent. Seizures that can be related to nervous system problems other than head trauma will recur within 20 months in 28 percent of cases. The risk of recurrence is not substantially affected by the prescription of anticonvulsant medication, but this may be because individuals who have had only one seizure often stop taking the medication after a few weeks.

LONG-TERM TREATMENT. Both parents and children often ask if the drugs used to control the seizures can be stopped. The side effects of the anticonvulsant may interfere with the child's social acceptance, and so the patient hopes to discontinue the drugs as early as possible. Some types of childhood seizure disorders are clearly self-limiting. For example, by the end of adolescence the child with benign Rolandic seizures of childhood will be seizure-free. With this type of seizure disorder, the family can be told not only that the medication can be stopped, but also when. Obviously, if a child has poorly controlled seizures while on anticonvulsants, it is not appropriate to stop the drugs. The true dilemma arises when a child's seizures have been completely controlled for several years. Fortunately there are empirical guidelines for deciding what to do.

If there is no apparent explanation for the seizures, even if the patient has focal neurologic abnormalities, the risk of seizures recurring is 26 percent once three seizure-free years have passed. If the patient had earlier neurologic injury from, say, meningitis or a head injury, the risk of recurrence goes up to 34 percent after three seizure-free years.

After four years without seizures on anticonvulsant medication, a child has a 72 percent chance of remaining seizure-free for decades if he stops taking the anticonvulsant. Of the 28 percent who have renewed seizure activity after going off the drugs, 85 percent will have the relapse within the first five years and 56 percent will have the relapse in the first year. The risk of relapse is greatest if the child had several years of poor seizure control before control was finally achieved, if there is unequivocal central nervous system damage associated with the seizures, if the child had jacksonian or other types of focal motor seizures, or if the child has had more than one type of epilepsy. Children with a history of a febrile seizure followed by a nonfebrile seizure also run a substantial risk of recurrent seizures when medication is discontinued.

With certain types of seizures, spontaneous remission is very likely. Of children whose electroencephalograms show no abnormality except in the brain waves arising from the occipital lobe, 48 percent will be seizure-free by the time they reach 9 years of age. The actual number of seizures the patient had before control was achieved does not affect the likelihood that he will remain seizure-free without medication. The age of the child when medication is stopped is also not important in determining the likelihood of remission, unless the seizures resisted control for several years before the child became seizure-free. The age at onset of the epilepsy, the sex of the child, and a family history of epilepsy also do not affect the likelihood of remaining seizure-free, even though some of these factors do influence the likelihood that a single seizure will develop into epilepsy. Once a seizure disorder has become established and seizures have been controlled with antiepileptic drugs, relapse is not more frequent in children with persistently abnormal electroencephalograms, so these cannot be used as an indication of the probability of remission. The patients with the best chance of remaining seizure-free without medication after four years of complete control are those with generalized, that is, grand mal and petit mal, seizures. Although generalized tonic-clonic (grand mal) seizures have always been viewed with the most horror by the parents of epileptic children, they actually have a relatively good prognosis.

Mortality

Premature death in children with epilepsy is not a real problem, although it is a preoccupation with many parents. When the first seizure occurs, many parents believe that their child is dying. This panic hardly subsides as the seizures become more routine. There are certain progressive diseases of the nervous system that cause seizures and are lethal during childhood, but the seizures associated with these diseases are not the cause of death. Even among patients whose epilepsy starts in adolescence, there is no excessive mortality.

The excess mortality that does occur in young people who have epilepsy without progressive brain disease is caused by status epilepticus, accidents, and suicide (see Chapter 10). Suicide attempts are not particularly common in children or adolescents, although by failing to take medication a patient may inadvertently risk death. Accidents are very common in epileptic children and adolescents, but in fatal accidents it is often impossible to determine if the epilepsy or the anticonvulsant medication played a role.[22]

Most children with epilepsy have normal intelligence, unimpaired growth, and conventional expectations. If a child's epilepsy is caused by a serious nervous system disturbance, this will usually be evident before or shortly after the appearance of the epilepsy. If it is a treatable lesion, the seizures may remit when it is corrected. If it is untreatable, the child's prognosis will be determined by the problem causing the seizures, not by the seizures themselves. Some types of epilepsy are not usually persistent: febrile seizures more often than not are benign and require no treatment other than management of the fever and the infection causing the fever; some types of nonfebrile childhood seizures, such as Rolandic seizures, are also benign and will disappear as the child matures. Before initiating treatment for any seizure, the physician must establish that the child actually does have epilepsy. Several benign conditions, such as breathholding spells and migraine, may resemble epilepsy, but careful neurologic assessment will determine which children have epilepsy and which do not.

Those children who do have epilepsy face a variety of social problems. They may be singled out at home and at school as distinctly different from their peers, and this assessment often becomes self-fulfilling. This stigmatizing of the epileptic child can be minimized if the parents and other family members have a clear idea of what the child can and cannot do. Relationships between the epileptic child and other members of his family must be flexible. As the child matures, what is expected of him and what is done for him must change.

Conflicts easily develop in a family with an epileptic child. Many of these can be avoided if all family members recognize the ease with which the child's epilepsy can add stress to the family. Power struggles between the affected child and other members of the family should be identified and stopped before manipulation becomes a way of life. The child should be allowed to face the usual challenges of childhood and should be allowed to fail.

Maturation does not necessarily resolve the problems caused by epilepsy; in fact it may present new ones. Adolescents with epilepsy are often just as impaired by the seizure disorder as they were in childhood, but they are often much less cooperative. One way to minimize the antagonism that appears between epileptic adolescents and their parents is gradually to give children more responsibility for their own activities and for managing their seizures. Using this approach, parents may ensure that when their children are most insistent on being independent they are adequately prepared to be independent.

Chapter 7

Children Growing
Up with an
Epileptic Parent

Patrick was born a year after his father developed epilepsy. The father's seizures were totally disabling, so he was usually at home, and Patrick was often present during seizures. When Patrick started crawling, he treated the seizures as a game. He would laugh during the falls and convulsions and even climb onto his father during some of the attacks. This amusement passed within a few months, and by his first birthday the child would cry when a seizure occurred and be agitated for hours afterwards. Despite his obvious discomfort with the attacks, the child stayed near his father during most of the day. His father noticed that Patrick was almost always with him when he had a seizure and always there when he awoke from a seizure.

Patrick started talking when he was about a year old, and his most common phrase was "He's okay," which he would say to his mother after his father had recovered from a seizure. During the early postictal period, the father would open his eyes and look around with obvious confusion. Patrick would stare at his father's face until the eyes opened and then announce, "He's okay, he's okay." When Patrick began speaking in fuller sentences, he would run to his mother when his father showed any signs of developing a seizure and tell her, "Daddy is sick again." By 18 months he could imitate the seizures with extraordinary accuracy. He would reenact facial expressions and limb postures that were part of the stereotyped motor phenomena preceding a generalized convulsion. He would fall to the ground, roll his eyes, and exhibit both the tonic and clonic phases of his father's seizures. This became a way to amuse friends; Patrick would imitate seizures at parties for his playmates. At one party a child was frightened by the seizure and told his mother, "I think Patrick is dead." Patrick opened his eyes and said, "I'm not dead. I'm just having a seizure."

Patrick also used the seizures to get attention. On a shopping trip with his parents, he saw a mechanical horse he wanted to ride. When his parents refused to let him, he had a pseudoseizure. Other shoppers, seeing him thrashing about on the floor, asked his apparently unconcerned parents if they could help. When one passerby demanded that the parents help the child with his seizure, Patrick announced, "I'm not having a real seizure. I just want to play on the horse." At the end of every pseudoseizure, Patrick would open his eyes and say, "I'm okay. I'm okay." His parents bought him a toy telephone, and he often pretended to call his father's doctor. His parents would overhear him saying, "Hello, Doctor Rothman. My daddy is okay today."

Whether parents try to conceal their epileptic attacks from their children or explain to the children that the epilepsy is not a sign of serious disease, children are usually aware of their parents' problem and feel considerable anxiety. The anxiety is apparent whether the child is a toddler or an adolescent. As was obvious in Patrick's case, knowing about the parent's epilepsy from the beginning does not necessarily make it less distressing.

How the young child understands the neurologic disorder is obviously influenced by the parents' attitudes; if the parents offer no explanation for what is happening, the child may develop an explanation that blames himself for causing the seizures. Part of the child's reaction is a fear of being abandoned; this is more of a preoccupation for toddlers and young children than for adolescents and young adults. Older children and adolescents worry about how their peers will view the parent's disorder. The notion that the epilepsy is hereditary or indicates a hereditary mental defect is pervasive enough that many children will conceal their parent's problem. Many children of epileptic parents worry that they will develop epilepsy.[1]

Learning about Epilepsy

Patrick learned about his father's seizures by seeing them occur. The postictal confusion, frequent injuries, and protracted fatigue associated with the seizures became as familiar to him as any element of his father's daily routine. Why he perceived these episodes as dangerous is not clear. His parents had married at about the same time as the first appearance of the seizures. Within a few months of the marriage it was obvious that the husband's episodic confusion was caused by a seizure disorder. The wife's resolve to have a successful marriage was unshaken by the revelation that her husband had epilepsy. Over the years she dealt with seizures calmly and consistently. She was not outwardly anxious during the attacks, and she allowed the child to watch the attacks so that he could see that nothing permanent was happening to his father. Patrick was an only child, so his anxiety was not based upon the reaction of older siblings. Friends and relatives who were present during some attacks did become very agitated, and this may have suggested to the child that something terrible was happening.

Although most people with epilepsy learn about the disorder from their physicians, and their spouses often ask the physician for information, the children of an epileptic parent usually find out about the disorder from one of their parents. The information they get is often distorted. The person with epilepsy usually does not absorb much of what he is told by his physician at the time of diagnosis, and he may be reluctant to ask detailed questions later, after months or years have passed. Basic questions such as "Is this epilepsy?" or "Can this be treated?" will be asked several times. Obviously, parents who are dazed by the news that they have a chronic illness are poor sources of information for their children. The spouse without epilepsy is rarely better prepared to explain the problem to the children. The parents may use ambiguous terms to describe the disorder, such as "drop attacks," "apoplexy," "blackouts," or "nervousness."

Many children are unaware that their parent has a seizure disorder until they witness an attack. When the child then is told that the problem has existed for years, he is likely to be skeptical and untrusting. Knowing that he has not been told the truth about his parent's health for years, he has little reason to believe he is now being given all the facts.

Without a reliable source of information in the family, the child will learn about the disorder from peers, television programs, and publications. These sources give the child no opportunity to clarify what his parent's problem is. Epilepsy is usually portrayed as a single entity, rather than as a collection of disorders. The child may get the impression that his parent's condition is much more serious and dangerous than it really is.

The child is at the greatest disadvantage if he is told nothing about the parent's disorder. Not only must he gather information from unreliable sources, but he must also search for explanations for why his parents are not willing to talk about the problem. The 7-year-old neighbor of a middle-aged man who had recently developed seizures asked if the man "would have to be put to sleep." The child had had a dog that had been put to sleep because of epilepsy, and as far as she knew, this was the way to treat the disorder. This type of information is what the child of an epileptic parent must contend with if the parents do not discuss the problem in terms the child can understand. If the parents make it clear that epilepsy is a topic the family can discuss, the misinformation provided by other children can be brought home and considered there.

Many children who are not fully informed about their parent's disorder will assume that a psychiatric problem or a more lethal illness is causing the trouble. One middle-aged physician with psychomotor seizures never told any of his four children that he had a seizure disorder. He insisted, "this does not affect them in any way. There's no reason to burden them with this." He maintained that, despite disruptive attacks, none of his family other than his wife and no one that he worked with suspected that he had epilepsy. Subsequently he had a seizure while driving with his youngest children in the car. They were unhurt but terrified. Still insisting that knowing about the epilepsy would only frighten them, he avoided any discussion about the accident and continued to drive as if this posed no danger for him or his children. Later he had another seizure while driving, and caused an accident. His youngest daughter, who was with him at the time of the accident, refused to ride with him after that, although he assured her that nothing was wrong. His children, forced to guess what the problem was, found their assumptions frightening enough to insist that their father not be responsible for their safety.

Fear of Abandonment

Seizures in a parent are frightening for children of any age, but young children have some very special fears. The most obvious concern of the young child is that the parent may abandon him. Whether the child actually witnesses the parent's attacks or only witnesses the responses of other family members, he invariably worries about losing the parent.[2]

There are several ways the child may react to this fear. Patrick became obsessed with his father's well-being and constantly monitored it. Another child, Robert, reacted with more alarm to his father's seizures, but also took on the role of monitor for the family. Robert was 3 when his father's seizures, a result of surgery the father had had before Robert was born, became poorly controlled. Over the course of a year Robert witnessed several seizures. Each time he cried uncontrollably and could not be comforted. After a seizure episode, he would stay awake most of the night. Several times he asked his mother, "Is Daddy going to die?" Despite reassurances from both of his parents, he insisted, "I'm sleeping with my daddy." Both parents described Robert as the "closest of all the children to his father." After his parents were in bed, Robert routinely knocked on the bedroom door and asked, "Daddy, are you okay?"

Transfer of Dependence

Children may assume considerable responsibility for the epileptic parent, but they too need someone to rely on. They sometimes shift their dependence from the adult with seizures to other family members. Laura, the teenage daughter of a woman who developed epilepsy late in life, showed considerable concern with her mother's health, but she relied on other members of her family for advice and assistance. Her mother developed seizures just as Laura was about to take a trip abroad, and Laura faced much conflict over whether to go. Her maternal aunt and grandfather insisted that she go. Over the next few years she continued to turn to her mother's sister for the kind of guidance that would ordinarily be provided by a parent. She remained quite attached to her mother, but she described her mother's illness as if she, rather than her mother, had suffered an injury. She said, "It was the worst thing that ever happened to me."

The shift away from dependence on the epileptic parent is probably reinforced by this feeling of injury. Laura's belief that the epilepsy was an injury to her is not at all unusual. David, an 11-year-old boy who did not know about his mother's lifelong generalized seizures until he witnessed one, became hysterical during the seizure. He hid and cried, and when his mother recovered he complained to her that it was not fair to him for her to be sick. He spoke of her illness as if it were terminal, insisting, "You can't be that sick. I didn't know you were so sick." His mother's epilepsy was actually easily controlled, and her seizure occurred only because of a lapse in medication combined with alcohol abuse. David felt that he had been tricked by not being told about her disease, and he refused to believe it was not lethal. His 14-year-old sister took the episode more stoically, but later in the day surprised her mother with the announcement, "You can't have this. You can't do this to me." In keeping with the family tradition of not discussing the epilepsy, both children refused to discuss the episode further and rejected the proposal that they visit the neurologist's office to have their questions answered.

The parent's seizures are a divisive element in some families. If the child is asked to watch the parent with epilepsy and report his or her behavior to the other parent, the family may split into two camps. The daughter of a middle-aged man with seizures was in the car when her father had an episode of altered consciousness and drove off the road. Because he did not want to give up driving, the girl lied to her mother about the accident. She insisted that her father had not had a seizure, even though she knew that a seizure had endangered both her and her father. By covering up for her father she established herself as an adversary to her mother, who sought to protect her husband by denying him activities he enjoyed.

Whether the child takes on responsibility for the epileptic parent or relies on another adult, the child does not consider the parent a dependable source of guidance and comfort. If the child learns about the seizures after the parents have concealed them for years, the parents lose credibility. The notion that a parent's seizure disorder is of no concern to the children is apparently not shared by the children once they discover the disorder.

Fears of Developing Epilepsy

Children of epileptic parents often fear that they will develop the disorder when they get older. This concern is evident whether the affected parent has idiopathic epilepsy or seizures secondary to a structural brain lesion. When the fear is appropriate, the child may exhibit an extraordinary level of denial. When a teenage girl whose father, brother, and grandfather had epilepsy first developed seizures, she refused to believe she had a permanent disorder. Despite having generalized convulsions with loss of consciousness at dangerous times, she refused to take anticonvulsant medications, insisting that she would grow out of the problem. She continued to have brief episodes of confusion for several years, but consistently denied that they were related to epilepsy. She lost personal items, including her wallet, and often could not remember how she had arrived home. When her problem was revealed to her father's neurologist, she stopped accompanying her parents to the doctor's office.[3]

Recommendations

The children of people with epilepsy show a remarkably limited range of reactions to the disorder. This simplifies the approach to these children, because it allows similar methods to be used in most situations. Regardless of the age of the child, the least disruptive approach to the parent's neurologic problem seems to be full disclosure. Unless the child is exceedingly unperceptive, he or she will notice the parent's altered consciousness, abnormal movements, or other seizure phenomena. If the seizures are fully controlled, the parent's chronic dependence on medication will arouse suspicion that a medical problem is involved. It is unrealistic to expect children to ask questions about a problem their parents refuse to discuss. Even when the problem is finally out in the open, children will still tend to stick to the pattern the family developed over the years. That is, they will avoid the topic with the same fervor exhibited by their parents.

Parents who are "found out" because they have a seizure are compromised in two respects. They are no longer viewed as physically reliable, and they lose their credibility. The child assumes that an illness justifying such secrecy must be grave. And the parent's reassurances that it is not serious are not believed, because the parent has been found untrustworthy. Frank discussion of the neurologic problem and its treatment can avoid the distrust and resentment that usually develop when the parents try to conceal the epilepsy. Because the parents may be burdened by their own misconceptions about the disorder, it is wise to involve a medical or mental health professional in at least some of the family discussions.

Chapter 8

Siblings and the Extended Family

Witnessing a seizure can be a frightening experience for the brother, sister, grandparent, or other relative of a person with epilepsy. The distress of relatives who see someone in the family have a seizure or who simply learn of the epilepsy often contributes to the isolation of the person with the disorder. Relatives are subject to the same prejudices and misconceptions about the neurologic disorder as anyone else in the general population. Finding out that a family member has epilepsy does not correct these misconceptions and may even solidify what had been vague concerns and fears.

When epilepsy occurs in a child, it may interfere with the development of constructive relationships between the child and the rest of the family. As brothers and sisters see the affected child receive special treatment or considerable attention, resentment is unavoidable. The adult who develops epilepsy also inevitably faces some deterioration in family ties. Why this alienation occurs so often is not obvious. The inaccurate information that relatives seem to accumulate certainly plays a role, but the compelling force driving most relatives away from the person with epilepsy is the fear that they will be obliged to help if a seizure occurs. It is upsetting enough to observe a seizure without having the added concern that the health or life of a loved one depends upon timely action. Most people do not know what to do if a seizure occurs and do not want to be in a situation where that knowledge might be essential. Nevertheless, they continue to burden the immediate family with useless, disturbing, and inaccurate information.

Who was responsible for the epilepsy often becomes one of the many absurd issues that divide the family. The often guilt-ridden person with epilepsy may find relatives reinforcing that gnawing sense of responsibility for the problem. Parents may burden a child with arguments over which of them was at fault. When the seizure disorder is idiopathic, the accusations often shift to which side of the family the problem was inherited from. Annoyed by these reactions, the person with epilepsy often welcomes the alienation from the rest of the family that eventually develops.

Fear and Denial

Relatives of a person with epilepsy often have an inordinate fear that they themselves will develop the disorder. This concern has some statistical validity, at least for the brothers and sisters of individuals with epilepsy. For 10 percent of the people who develop epilepsy, at least one sibling has a history of seizure disorders. If someone has had only one seizure, the risk that he will have other seizures is substantially greater if he has a brother or sister with epilepsy: for idiopathic seizures, 35 percent of the siblings who have one seizure will have another within four months if they have an epileptic brother or sister. This simply means that susceptibility to epilepsy, like susceptibility to allergies and heart disease, is greater in some families than in others. The sister of a child with idiopathic seizures will not necessarily develop epilepsy, but the probability that she will have seizures at some time in her life is slightly greater than that of other children in the general population.[1]

The fear experienced by children who witness epilepsy in a sibling may be quite disabling. Even children who have routinely been helpful and considerate with their siblings may find that the disorder terrifies them into paralysis. Paula developed generalized seizures when she was 14 years old. Although she was started on antiepileptic drugs shortly after the appearance of her first generalized tonic-clonic (grand mal) attack, she continued to have seizures about once a month. Her brother, Robert, three years younger, did not witness a convulsion until he was 12 years old. He and Paula were helping their father with household chores when Paula abruptly fell to the floor and began to convulse. The father asked Robert to get some pillows to put around Paula to keep her from hurting herself. Obviously terrified, Robert ran into his own room and lay in his bed trembling. Several minutes after his sister had recovered, he emerged from his room in tears. "I wanted to help," was all he could say.

Such paralysis occurs in adults as well. One young man with frequent seizures discovered that when he had a seizure his mother-in-law and sister-in-law started screaming and his sister abandoned him in terror without even volunteering to get help. This failure to be helpful is common in the family around a person with epilepsy, and it is a particularly divisive force. The wife of a young man with complex partial seizures recalled with irritation that her husband's sister waited out in the hallway at the hospital when he developed a generalized convulsion. The sister's inability to help during this incident was less irritating than her refusal to stay near enough to provide emotional support for the wife.

Family members often refuse to hear that the individual has epilepsy. A middle-aged man who developed epilepsy after an automobile accident made several attempts to tell his only brother that he had a seizure disorder, and with each attempt his brother turned the discussion to the weather, sports, or another irrelevant matter. His brother did not visit him in the hospital when a bout of frequent seizures obliged him to be admitted, and other relatives provided no comfort or aid to his family when his seizures were at their worst. This man could explain such callous behavior only by assuming, "They cannot conceive that I have a problem."

Fault-Finding and Resentment

One of the more pernicious roles played by an unhelpful family is making those closest to the epileptic person feel that they are not doing enough or that they are doing something wrong. The parents, spouses, and siblings of people with epilepsy all face a barrage of irrelevant and largely inaccurate information brought to them under the guise of helpfulness. To avoid this type of harassment, they may disavow all responsibility for control of the seizure disorder, placing it with another family member or the epileptic person himself. This response contributes to the isolation of the individual with epilepsy.

Some siblings act as if the disorder is contrived or self-serving. A watchman who was injured in a robbery attempt and had to undergo brain surgery was vexed by his sister's recurrent jibes that he was doing very nicely on his disability income, an income justified by his having as many as ten seizures daily. As a gift at one of the family's celebrations, she bought him a T-shirt that announced that he was a welfare recipient. By minimizing the epileptic person's problems, the family denies him the option of depending upon them. Although a small segment of the population with epilepsy does exploit the disability, the prejudice that anyone with this type of chronic disorder will exploit it is not justified by the facts.

Some patients with epilepsy claim that brothers, sisters, and other members of the family take the disorder personally. They react as if the epileptic person purposely has the neurologic problem to upset them. Implicit in this reaction is the feeling that the individual with epilepsy is at least partly responsible for his problem. A young mother whose son temporarily lost consciousness after a head injury was worried that the boy might have the seizure disorder her own brother had developed in childhood. She described her brother as generally incompetent and careless. That he had epilepsy and that he had failed to achieve any social goals considered significant by his family were intimately tied together in his sister's view of him. She had little to do with him, largely because she considered him responsible for his poor seizure control. As she saw it, he had not taken charge of his life.

This is not an unusual view for the family to take of the individual with epilepsy, and it is often accurate. But this perception ignores the special obligations faced by the epileptic person. People unburdened by epilepsy are not obliged to constantly monitor their own behavior and take medication. What the family often sees is someone living in the careless manner in which they all live, but suffering special consequences.

Constructive Approaches

When a child has epilepsy, it is important to give the nonepileptic siblings their share of parental attention and to recognize their limitations. They should not be required to help manage the epileptic child's seizures or to provide emotional support for their parents. The epileptic child's brothers and sisters face their own problems and have a right to the same help that parents give the child with epilepsy.

When an adult has epilepsy, the friction in the immediate and extended family must be minimized, and some of the burden of achieving this invariably falls upon the person with the seizures. Much of what seems like malice or insensitivity in family members is nothing more than denial of a frightening condition, the epilepsy. Relatives who do not have the problem cannot truly understand what the person with epilepsy must face every day, and they should not be expected to understand. By ignoring what could easily be taken as abrasive remarks and behavior, the person with epilepsy may be able to preserve family relationships that will prove invaluable over the course of a lifetime.

Chapter 9

Personality Changes and Violence

What happens to the thoughts, behavior, personality, mood, and other psychologic aspects of people with epilepsy has been disputed for decades. Some physicians have insisted that none of these brain functions are altered by seizure activity, and others have claimed that specific defects may appear in individuals with specific types of epilepsy. The controversy is far from being settled. What may be said with some confidence is that many people exhibit no change in thoughts, feelings, or actions as a direct result of the seizure disorder, but that many others do have psychologic changes associated with particular types of epilepsy. This does not necessarily mean that the psychologic changes are caused by the epilepsy itself. These changes and the seizure disorder may simply be two manifestations of one nervous system disease or injury.

Problems with mood and behavior develop in people with epilepsy at least as often as in people with other chronic diseases. Depression and anger are appropriate and unavoidable when the seizure disorder is poorly controlled or when treatment measures are causing problems of their own. However, some individuals with epilepsy exhibit more disruptive behavior than can be attributed to depression. Some of this behavior is undeniably violent and may have tragically damaging consequences. Violent behavior occasionally occurs during the ictus of the seizure, but most of it happens during postictal confusion. There remains, however, in a small segment of the population with epilepsy, much peculiar and some truly sociopathic behavior that is unrelated to specific seizures.

Opinions differ widely about the relationship between these personality changes, violent behavior, and particular seizure disorders, but the consensus is that purposely violent behavior is not characteristic of any type of epilepsy. Aggressive, destructive behavior during a seizure has been clearly documented in very few instances. Individuals with epilepsy certainly may damage property or injure people who try to subdue them while they are confused or convulsing, but this type of destructiveness is obviously not intentional. After the seizure proper, the victim may still be too confused to act coherently for several minutes or even hours and may cause what appears to be much more intentional damage. This is not the most common type of behavior in the postictal period, a period during which most people are lethargic and confused, but neither is it extremely rare.[1]

Personality Traits

Fewer than 25 percent of patients with seizure disorders are free of any intellectual, behavioral, or simply neurologic problems. About 50 percent have significant psychological or social problems that show up in their daily activities and behavior. Depression, excessive anxiety, self-denigration, hypochondriasis, confused thinking, excessive sensitivity, and a pervasive dissatisfaction are commonly reported by and observed in adults with epilepsy. That is not to say that everyone who has epilepsy has these problems; in fact, an epileptic individual is most likely to have several or none of these traits. These are not abnormal personality traits in any sense, but they do interfere with normal activities when they are persistent.[2]

Many people with epilepsy are embarrassed when their seizures occur, feel considerable resentment that they have this problem at all, feel that their worth is diminished because of the disorder, and occasionally feel less accepted by others because of their condition. Again, none of these feelings is abnormal, and in fact 70 percent of those with epilepsy feel neither unreasonably limited nor subject to special treatment because of their seizures.[3]

Unquestionable psychologic problems and changes are most

common in patients with complex partial epilepsy, especially in those whose seizures first appear during adolescence. Developing epilepsy before or after adolescence results in a lower overall rate of personality disorders, an observation that is not explained by current notions on the evolution of seizures. This phenomenon may occur because of a special vulnerability in adolescence to problems that interfere with the development of a stable self-image.[4]

Although substantial psychologic problems in people with idiopathic seizures are fairly uncommon, some patients with complex partial (psychomotor) seizures have problems ranging from hyperactive behavior and violence to sexual dysfunction and hypochondriasis. Schizophrenia and psychotic depressions are rare in people with epilepsy, but they appear more frequently in patients with complex partial seizures than in those with any other type of epilepsy. This observation reinforces the impression that patients with seizures originating in damaged structures in the temporal lobe of the brain are particularly vulnerable to psychiatric disorders.[5]

Obsessive and paranoid traits are especially characteristic of people whose seizures originate in the temporal lobe and develop before puberty. The paranoid ideas these people have are often religious or mystical in character. Some have multiple religious conversions after mystical experiences. God speaks to them directly and tells them what religion to practice and preach. In addition to having this feeling of a divine importance or a religious mission, these patients often ascribe great significance to commonplace events. A book that accidentally falls open will be seen as a warning or a prophecy. A fellow worker's cough may be interpreted as a criticism. Inconsequential events will be recorded in detailed diaries as part of a compulsion to write down everything.[6]

In many instances, the personality changes that occur when someone develops epilepsy are neither peculiar nor undesirable. A family may notice that a previously abusive member has mellowed with the evolution of the seizure disorder. An embarrassingly reserved member of the family may become more outgoing. These kinds of changes in personality obviously do not require treatment. When a serious personality disorder develops, however, and when treatment of the seizures alone does not correct it, psychiatric intervention may be necessary.

Mood Disturbances

The depression and other mood disturbances experienced by some people with epilepsy are more than just reactions to poor seizure control. The incidence of serious depressions in people with epilepsy has remained largely unchanged over the past thirty years despite substantial advances in seizure control. Serious mood disturbances are not limited to patients who require hospitalization for frequent seizures or other neurologic problems; 17 to 25 percent of people with epilepsy who are not hospitalized have psychologic problems that interfere with their daily functioning, and at least 10 percent need psychiatric intervention or hospitalization at some time in their lives. A suicide attempt is often the reason for the psychiatric attention. This self-destructive bent is not just a response to chronic disability, since the people with epilepsy who have the most severe mood disturbances are often much less disabled than people with other chronic medical problems who exhibit no mood disorders. The severity of the mood disorder does not parallel the severity of the seizure disorder.[7]

What is a persistent mood disorder and what is simply another facet of the seizure disorder is not always obvious. Some patients, especially those whose seizures originate in the temporal lobe, develop overwhelming fear with the seizures or between seizure episodes. Because it is part of the seizure proper (the ictus), this is usually called ictal fear. It is the most common emotion felt during seizures, and it is experienced by as many as 22 percent of those with temporal lobe origins for the epilepsy. The evaluation of this baseless emotion is complicated by the appearance of a more abiding fear in many of these patients, a fear that lasts for hours or days between the obvious seizure episodes.[8]

Treating mood disturbances with antidepressant drugs poses special problems for people with epilepsy. Many antidepressants, such as the tricyclic compounds imipramine (Tofranil) and amitriptyline (Elavil), lower the seizure threshold and may be particularly dangerous for depressed patients who might ignore instructions on how to take the medication. To treat severe depression in patients without seizure disorders, the physician has the option of using electroconvulsive therapy. In epileptic patients, however, this is even more dangerous than antidepressants, because what this shock technique induces is nothing more than a seizure. Both pharmaceutical and electroshock approaches to the depression carry the risk of exacerbating the seizure disorder. This does not mean that the depression, anxiety, or fear experienced by these patients should not be treated; what it means is that drugs or electroconvulsive therapy must be applied with constant attention to the increased risk of seizures. To leave these severe mood disturbances untreated is to run the risk of suicide.

Violent Behavior

The damage done by an epileptic person during and shortly after a seizure is random and gives the person neither personal gain nor satisfaction. In fact, much of the damage may be inflicted upon items the person specifically tries to protect. A vase pushed out of the way in the last confused moment before a generalized convulsion may be broken; a child inadvertently placed on a precarious support during the altered perceptions of a partial seizure may be injured. Inadvertent destructiveness is most common in the postictal period.[9]

Deciding whether the damage is intentional is also most difficult during the postictal period. The patient may seem fully alert and aware of what he or she is doing and may make threats that seem too well-conceived to be the ranting of a confused mind. Even the amnesia or imperfect recall of events during this violent period is difficult for witnesses to believe, partly because there is a seamless transition from the confusion and irritability of the postictal period to the clarity and remorse of the interictal period. It is understandable that onlookers think the disorganized aggressiveness results from malicious intent, but in fact the damage is done because of confusion rather than malice or anger. The anger may appear authentic, but the justifications for it are illogical or delusional. Individuals who can remember even fragments of the seizure after it is over are routinely embarrassed and remorseful.

Violent behavior during a seizure is occasionally a reaction to well-formed delusions or hallucinations, which may result from a tumor or other physical problem in the brain (Figure 9.1). Patients may react to their threatening hallucinations with outbursts directed toward real people around them. A cup of coffee in someone's hand may be seen as a gun. A casual greeting may be heard as an angry threat. The victim of the seizure reacts to these menacing delusions with terror or violence. This ictal violence can be more dangerous than the postictal confusion and irritability that accounts for most sociopathic behavior in individuals with epilepsy, but the violence is too random and too disorganized to cause much real injury to anyone except the epileptic victim himself.

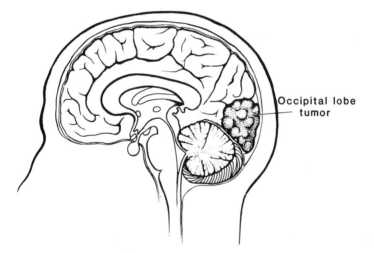

Figure 9.1 Tumor overlying the brain. A person with hallucinations may have a psychiatric problem, but occasionally hallucinations are caused by structural lesions in or on the brain. A tumor pressing on the occipital lobe can cause focal sensory seizures that are mistaken for delusions or hallucinations.

The belief that criminal activities can be the result of epileptic seizures has been reinforced by the increasing number of pleas in criminal court alleging that a defendant accused of an aggressive, violent, or simply felonious act was having a seizure at the time. The argument is that the defendant cannot be held responsible for the crime because when the crime was committed he was suffering from altered consciousness imposed by the epilepsy. Complex partial epilepsy is the seizure disorder most often invoked as the basis for the altered mental state, but most neurologists do not believe that repeated violence and destructive behavior can be ascribed to this or any seizure type. People with epilepsy may commit robbery, assault, rape, or murder, but not because they have epilepsy. They commit crimes for the same reasons that people without epilepsy commit crimes. Criminal intent does not develop from the epilepsy.[10]

Relationship of Violence to Seizure Type

Many studies have suggested that violence associated with epilepsy is most likely to occur if the victim of the seizure disorder has complex partial epilepsy, but the findings in this area have been very inconsistent. There clearly are many patients in epilepsy clinics with seizures arising from temporal lobe damage who have obvious mental illness, peculiar social behavior, or unusual personality traits. A few of these patients have frank psychoses, some have personality disorders that keep them from developing relationships or being gainfully employed, and some exhibit clearly violent or destructive behavior. But these clinic patients are quite atypical of people with epilepsy. They are usually indigent, have poor seizure control, and exhibit numerous social problems. Highly compliant, socially integrated people with well-controlled epilepsy are less likely to be in the clinic group; they do not require regular supervision. These considerations aside, there is little consistent evidence that criminal behavior occurs more often in victims of complex partial seizures than in patients with generalized tonic-clonic (grand mal) seizures or, for that matter, in the general population.[11]

Studies that have linked complex partial seizures with aggressive, destructive, or otherwise sociopathic behavior have been primarily preoperative or postoperative evaluations of patients with intractable seizures treated surgically. In these patients, definite structural damage to the temporal lobe is found in 80 percent of cases, a relatively high rate of pathology for a population of individuals with epilepsy. Aggressive behavior is the most common psychologic problem described, but this is manifested by unpredictable outbursts of anger during the interictal period. Although children with temporal lobe epilepsy alone do not have unprovoked attacks of rage, the individuals with epilepsy most likely to show irrational destructive or abusive behavior as adults are those whose seizures start early in childhood. When the anterior temporal lobe is surgically removed, the aggressive behavior disappears for more than six years in 20 percent of the patients so treated.[12]

Although much attention has been paid to aggressive or destructive behavior in people with temporal lobe damage or seizures that appear to originate in the temporal lobes, the current consensus leans away from any clear association between damage to the temporal lobe and sociopathic behavior. Even those who suggest that there is a causal relationship between temporal lobe epilepsy and aggression in some patients recognize that most patients with this type of epilepsy are not unusually aggressive. Male sex, low IQ, lack of religious ties, and juvenile behavior problems are all more important factors than epilepsy in the appearance of violent or destructive behavior disorders in people with epilepsy. Of the people with epilepsy who do exhibit aggressive behavior, 41 percent have a history of permanent separation from one or both parents before the age of 15. For many of these patients, it is disruptive behavior, rather than seizures, at an early age that initially brings them to medical attention. The patient's age at the onset of the seizure disorder may be important in the development of aggressive behavior, but even this is controversial.[13]

A complicating factor is that much of what is interpreted as psychopathology may be fairly routine postictal signs of a neurological disturbance. Patients whose seizures originate in the temporal lobes may have problems with word-finding during the interictal period. Presumably this is nothing more than a sign of disturbed temporal lobe function persisting long after obvious seizure activity has abated. Much of the peculiar behavior attributed to individuals with temporal lobe seizures may be caused by similar interictal disturbances.[14]

In children with complex partial epilepsy originating in the temporal lobes, episodes of rage and hyperactive behavior may occur when the seizures first develop. Although these episodes become less frequent as the child becomes an adult, recurrent depression becomes more of a problem. Some adults with complex partial epilepsy are remarkably irritable and have profound mood swings.[15]

John developed complex partial epilepsy when he was 45 years old. Before the disorder appeared he was always even-tempered and never raised his voice, used obscenities, or exhibited any violent behavior. "If the ceiling fell down next to him," his wife said, "he'd simply get up and move his chair." But as his seizures progressed from minor changes in consciousness to long spells of confusion with peculiar gestures and a tendency to wander, violent outbursts became routine. When some teenagers did not move out of his way as he was trying to park, he raced his car toward them, shouting obscenities at them as they jumped aside. When a woman tried to push ahead of him at a supermarket, he picked up her groceries and flung them to the ground. When his family questioned him about his violent behavior, he denied it and became abusive toward them. The abusiveness never occurred during a seizure or during the postictal period, but his wife noticed that his most violent episodes would be followed within hours by a seizure.

What may be most important in determining whether a person with complex partial epilepsy has violent or sociopathic outbursts is the type of damage that has occurred in the temporal lobe, rather than the type of seizure exhibited. The abnormal personality traits, the changes in personality, and the seizure activity may all be separate manifestations of a problem in the brain, rather than being causally related to one another.

Comparing episodes of violent behavior in patients with complex partial epilepsy and those with generalized epilepsy, some physicians find no relationship between the incidence of aggression and the seizure type. In those with generalized seizures, patients who are younger or who have myoclonic seizures are less likely to be violent than older patients with tonic-clonic seizures. Patients with akinetic seizures, a type of generalized seizure in which the affected individual temporarily stops all movement except breathing, have a clearly increased incidence of violent behavior.[16]

What does occur frequently in individuals with complex partial epilepsy is episodic abusiveness to family members. This is a problem for adults and is occasionally manifest as wife beating or husband beating. These violent outbursts are unrelated to apparent seizure episodes, but may be related to the overall level of seizure control.

Episodic Dyscontrol

Concern that aggressive criminal behavior might result from focal brain lesions has prompted considerable study of changes in aggression and violence after lesions in selected areas of the brain. The results of these studies, as well as the procedures used, are controversial. One problem is that often aggressive populations are studied to determine whether they show an unusually high incidence of epilepsy. A better method would be to start with a population of individuals known to have seizures and then to determine if this group shows an excess of destructive behavior. Even though some studies of prison populations have suggested that epilepsy is common in sociopathic individuals, the people usually studied have questionable evidence of seizure activity. More objective studies do not support the notion that epilepsy is a common basis for criminal behavior. According to fairly reliable studies from England, the prevalence of epilepsy is only slightly greater in prison populations than in the general population.[17]

Research on violent individuals and criminal populations has yielded the notion that a disorganized emotional or intellectual state is involved in many violent acts. This has been called the episodic dyscontrol syndrome. Individuals with this syndrome have discrete bouts of violent behavior that last minutes or hours. These paroxysms are largely unprovoked and are occasionally preceded by abnormal sensations. After an episode the individual often complains of headache or drowsiness. Implicit in the grouping of these behavior disorders into a syndrome is that a common nervous system disorder, perhaps an epileptic disorder, underlies the violence.

People with episodic dyscontrol share several characteristics besides their violent behavior. They are usually from poor families, have little formal education, and exhibit sociopathic behavior by their twenties or early thirties. Their fathers often are chronic alcoholics and child-abusers. More than 70 percent of those who develop episodic dyscontrol as adults are hyperactive in childhood, and half claim to have had staring spells, unrelated to violent behavior, that lasted seconds and involved "altered consciousness." These people are very remorseful, and about 50 percent claim that they have tried to kill themselves. Alcohol increases the frequency and severity of their criminal outbursts. More than 30 percent admit to sexual problems, including impotence, transvestitism, and obsessive abstinence from sex.

The episode of uncontrolled violence may be preceded by visual illusions, altered hearing, nausea, or pins-and-needles sensations. After the attack, some individuals claim that they do not remember what happened. Those that recall it deny that they could control it. Actually, these claims are fairly common for people accused of committing crimes: 72 percent of juveniles accused of committing violent crimes claim memory lapses, blackouts, dizziness, and dreamlike states during the crime and fatigue after the crime. These phenomena are probably subjective changes associated with excitement, rather than epilepsy.

On the assumption that epilepsy might be playing a role in these violent outbursts, some individuals with episodic dyscontrol were treated with antiepileptic drugs. Sixty-eight percent reported some improvement while on phenytoin. This is probably not significant, since the syndrome usually disappears on its own as the person gets older. Episodic dyscontrol rarely appears in anyone over 50 years of age. Evidence that epilepsy is an important or constant element in this syndrome is obviously weak. One reason the term episodic dyscontrol syndrome has had some popularity is that it does not label this behavior disorder as epilepsy.

Any objective study of violent individuals is complicated by what these people have to gain if they can convince a court of law that their underlying problem is epilepsy. Studies that show an incidence of epilepsy in prison populations ten times as high as in the general population are misleading. With the curious acceptance of epilepsy as a cause of violent behavior, a defense based on a nervous system disorder is likely to be offered in court. Unfortunately, the diagnosis of epilepsy in most cases relies heavily on the patient's own testimony, and so an excessive number of epileptic cases are discovered during trials. Many of these accused people admit that alcohol or other drugs played a role in their destructive behavior, and this too argues against their having epilepsy, since alcohol is an anticonvulsant. Episodic dyscontrol syndrome is probably a somewhat consistent personality disorder appearing in criminals.

Fugue States

In some types of epilepsy, the patient may enter a protracted trance-like state. This is an extremely rare situation, but it does occur in generalized absence (petit mal) and complex partial (psychomotor) seizures. This is called a fugue state, a term more commonly used to refer to episodes of wandering seen in individuals with schizophrenia or other psychoses. Patients with fugue states caused by epilepsy may be much less mobile and self-sufficient than patients with schizophrenic episodes, and their protracted episodes of confusion are also called twilight states if they appear to be part of the postictal period.

During the epileptic fugue state the patient has seizure activity that can be demonstrated with electrical studies of the brain. An electroencephalogram performed during the confused state will reveal diffuse electrical changes characteristic of seizure activity (see Chapter 10). After the episode the patient will generally not remember what happened. During the fugue or twilight state the patient will not be able to perform complex activities. When those patients travel, they get lost. If they are not given shelter, they stay exposed. In fugue and twilight states it is remarkable that the patient is conscious and active at all. Their activities usually do not appear normal. Someone encountering an individual in this condition would suspect that something was profoundly wrong. Amnesia is a relatively minor aspect of the fugue or twilight state.

Wife Beating, Husband Beating, and Child Abuse

When violent behavior does occur in a person with epilepsy, family members are often the targets. Family members are usually injured because they attempt to deal with the person having seizures as if he or she were perfectly rational and coherent. The wife, husband, or child trying hardest to cope with the epileptic person's erratic behavior is at the greatest risk.

Although abusiveness is often an obvious consequence of seizure activity, some patients exhibit abusive behavior that seems unconnected to seizures. When the abusiveness is largely unprovoked, lack of seizure control should be considered an important factor in the behavior and suppression of the seizures should be the first objective of treatment.

Abusive behavior need not occur during the seizure to be clearly related to seizure activity. One wife noticed that her husband would go through three typical stages before a seizure episode. He would become depressed, then increasingly irritable and verbally abusive, and then he would develop unequivocal seizures. In his irritable stage he repeatedly interfered with his wife's attempts to get medical help for him. This man did not physically abuse his wife, but another man with a similar pattern of progressive irritability consulted physicians specifically because he was beating his wife. After their seizures, both men were remorseful, but their wives doubted their sincerity and were afraid of them. For both men, improved seizure control resulted in less violent behavior. But the best way to decrease a patient's violence varies with specific features of each patient's disorder.

When a husband, wife, child, or parent becomes threatening

and abusive, family members should assume that the episode is irrational and potentially dangerous. Whether this outburst occurs during the ictus of a seizure, in the postictal period, or between seizures, direct confrontation with the violent person should be avoided. Trying to restrain a violent person during the postictal period risks substantial injury to both the victim of the epilepsy and the would-be helper. If an epileptic person becomes violent when a seizure has not occurred, family members should take this as a signal to keep their contact with that person at a minimum.

For any person who shows a tendency to violent behavior, firearms should be made inaccessible. Allowing someone with this problem to keep guns near at hand is foolish. Many family members believe they must stay nearby during the violent episodes as a sign of their trust. This type of behavior ignores the seizure victim's impaired condition and invites tragedy. If the patient's violent episodes endanger himself and family members might be injured in trying to protect him, the family should seek outside assistance. If the degree of confusion and potential for injury is relatively slight, an emergency ambulance crew or other paramedical professionals should be able to manage the situation. If the violence is more substantial, police intervention may be necessary. The family's first responsibility is to avoid tragedy, not to avoid embarrassment or hurt feelings.

Violence with Improved Seizure Control

With some seizure disorders, such as complex partial epilepsy, the patient may show increasingly violent behavior as the seizures are better controlled. A 40-year-old man with poorly controlled seizures was started on carbamazepine after having seizures more than once a month for several years. With this medication his seizures recurred much less often, but he found himself flying into rages. He broke furniture and beat his wife. She was terrified by his abrupt change in behavior and sought additional medical help. Rather than allowing him to have seizures and become more subdued, the physician increased the anticonvulsants to make him completely seizure-free and added antidepressant medication. With this change in drugs, the patient became less depressed, less violent, and free of seizures, but his wife was still afraid of him. Whenever he looked irritable, she would try to avoid his company. Although his violence had been transient, it caused a lasting rift in their marriage.

For many patients with complex partial seizures and violent outbursts, the outbursts seem to follow long seizure-free intervals. The abusive behavior lasts hours to days and may end abruptly when a seizure occurs. During this irritable period, the patient resists all efforts to calm him and broods over imagined slights or insults. Serious injury to others during this period is unlikely, and when the anger abates the patient is usually remorseful and apologetic. He remembers how he behaved and may promise to avoid such behavior in the future. Of course, the promise is forgotten when the next imagined slight provokes another episode of anger.

Because control of the seizure disorder may increase the frequency of the episodes, some physicians allow their patients to remain incompletely controlled if violent behavior between seizures is a problem. Allowing recurrent seizures is risky, because injury to the patient or status epilepticus may result. Combining treatment of the seizures with antipsychotic medications is a safer approach, but this type of therapy is only wise when the patient's violence is endangering family members or others.[18]

It is worth noting that much of the violence observed in patients whose seizures originate in the temporal lobes abates after surgery. This fact has been offered as a justification for using temporal lobe surgery to deal with violent behavior itself. But the long-term effects of the surgery are controversial and the cause of the observed changes is poorly understood. This type of surgery cannot be considered as a way of managing violent behavior (see Chapter 11).

Suicide Attempts

Self-destructive behavior is common in people with epilepsy. It may range from inappropriate risk-taking to unequivocal suicide attempts. Depression often accompanies any unremitting, chronic problem, but in some types of epilepsy the disorder itself probably contributes to the mood disturbance that leads to self-destructive behavior. Unfortunately, patients with seizure disorders have ready access to dangerous medications. Sometimes these drugs can contribute to a lethal outcome even if the patient does not intend to commit suicide. For example, driving a car when seizure control is poor is dangerous under the best of circumstances, but especially so when dosages of anticonvulsant drugs have recently been changed, because the change in medication may slow the patient's reaction times.[19]

Attempted suicide is common among patients with all types of epilepsy. Along with lethal events that are a direct expression of the disorder, such as untreated status epilepticus and seizure-related accidents, suicide ranks as a leading cause of death in people with epilepsy. As in any population of patients, there is also a group whose cause of death appears to be accidental or is never described as anything more than an unexplained cardiac arrest. The high incidence of accidental and unexplained deaths among the epileptic population suggests that the true incidence of suicide may be even higher than has been documented.

Some studies attribute 12 to 20 percent of deaths in individuals with epilepsy to suicide—five times the rate of attempted suicide in the general population (32.5 per thousand). The rate of suicide attempts among those with complex partial epilepsy may be as much as 25 times greater than that of the general population.

Two factors place patients with epilepsy at special risk: they have a high incidence of depressive illnesses, and they have easy access to nonviolent instruments of suicide, namely anticonvulsant drugs. Of those with epilepsy who attempt suicide, 84 percent try to poison or overdose themselves, and 65 percent use anticonvulsants. Overdoses of phenobarbital have always been especially popular; the respiratory depressant action of phenobarbital is often purposely enhanced by alcohol. About two-thirds of those who attempt suicide by self-poisoning take an anticonvulsant they have been prescribed, and another 15 percent combine their anticonvulsants with other drugs. Even though phenobarbital is being supplanted by other anticonvulsants, many of the antiepileptic medications in use are metabolized to phenobarbital, and others can depress breathing even though they are not barbiturates. When medication is closely supervised, the suicide rate is lower: patients in hospitals or other institutions are much less likely to commit suicide than are patients with epilepsy outside such facilities.

Men with epilepsy are more likely to attempt suicide than women with epilepsy; both men and women are more inclined to make serious suicide attempts when they are unemployed. Sixty percent of those with seizure disorders who attempt suicide are under 30 years of age. Repeated attempts are twice as common in people with epilepsy as in people without epilepsy: 74 percent of patients with seizures who fail in a suicide attempt will try again. Obviously the patient at greatest risk of repeated suicide attempts is the one who fails through misinformation alone. A patient who takes a massive dose of phenytoin and suffers little more than difficulty in walking, blurred vision, nausea, and vomiting may try again with a more effective drug. Careful observation and aggressive treatment of such patients is important in any plan to avert suicide.

Major psychiatric disorders, such as schizophrenia and manic-depressive (bipolar) psychoses, are no more common in suicidal individuals with epilepsy than in those without epilepsy, but there is a higher incidence of personality disorders in suicidal individuals with epilepsy. Epileptic patients face special social problems because of their chronic disorder, and sometimes they have the added disadvantage of personality disorders that limit their ability to cope with their unusual burdens. All this contributes to frustration and anger that may make the individual self-destructive.

To reduce the risk of future suicide attempts, the family and physician must consider the events leading to the self-destructive action. Multiple problems usually contribute to the patient's hopelessness, but there is often a distressing incident or an unresolvable problem that triggers the final dramatic gesture or sincere attempt at self-destruction. Some people fall into despair out of profound guilt over being constantly dependent or sick. One woman with epilepsy tried to kill herself because she felt responsible for her daughter's epilepsy. Problems with seizure control or difficulty in keeping a job are often given as reasons for suicide attempts, but the true reasons may be more subtle. For example, conflict with a spouse over financial worries or problems with seizure control may be more important in precipitating a suicide attempt than the unemployment or the seizure activity.

Self-Destructive Behavior through Noncompliance

A patient's decision to stop taking anticonvulsants may bring on the sometimes lethal convulsive disorder called status epilepticus. Although such potentially dangerous behavior as refusing medication is generally not included in statistics on suicide, it probably accounts for as much morbidity and mortality as do outright suicide attempts. A person with epilepsy can inflict considerable self-injury with minimal effort and planning.

Equally dangerous is a refusal to comply with restrictions on activity. Swimming, driving a car, rock climbing, and commuting by subway can all pose substantial threats to a person whose seizures are poorly controlled. Men especially resist giving up these prerogatives, which seem to be tied to their self-images. One patient insisted on driving when his family took trips even though others in the car could drive. He explained this as a way of testing himself. Ironically, when his activities did not threaten the safety of his entire family, he rarely insisted on driving. He seemed to cling to his role in the family more than to his own image of himself as a driver.

Minimizing Risks

To avoid tragedy, the epileptic individual and the family must recognize that the risk of self-injury exists. Allowing a family member with poorly controlled seizures to drive a car while the family is in it is a denial of risk that can be lethal for the entire family. Most states allow people with epilepsy to drive if they have been seizure-free for 12 months, whether or not they require medication. This is a reasonable position for the family to adopt in dealing with a member with epilepsy who is inclined to disregard the law.

When people with epilepsy are depressed, nothing is gained by leaving them to "work it out on their own." Problems, conflicts, and concerns should be explored with a psychotherapist or a physician familiar with the patient. Self-destructive behavior should not be ignored. Anything resembling a suicide attempt should immediately be brought to the physician's attention. Depression can be effectively treated, and the risks of self-destructive behavior can be minimized, but only if the problem is managed energetically and intelligently by experienced professionals. A suicide attempt is not something to be dealt with by sympathetic remarks over the dinner table. A therapist or physician should be involved in treating the depression.

Chapter 10

Investigating the Person with Epilepsy

Before epilepsy can be properly treated, it must be recognized. And even after it has been recognized, its cause remains to be established. Some seizure disorders, such as grand mal epilepsy, are obvious after only one attack, but others may not be suspected for weeks or months. The infant who has a generalized tonic-clonic seizure with a high fever will be quickly brought to a physician by the horrified parents. The same parents may observe several dozen staring spells or drop attacks before they suspect that their child has a medical problem. If they do not perceive the problem for some time, the gaps in the child's consciousness may interfere with learning and comprehension, and the child may even be mistakenly diagnosed as mentally retarded.[1]

Adults for whom bedwetting is the only symptom of generalized seizures may conceal their problem for years before mentioning it to a physician, and even then the physician may investigate them only from a urological—rather than a neurological—standpoint. Older adults with bedwetting in their sleep are often considered prematurely senile; epilepsy is suspected by neither the patient nor the family. An elderly person who loses consciousness during the day may be misconstrued as having had a stroke, which some people incorrectly believe to be a reasonable consequence of senility. This misinterpretation of increasing seizure activity leaves the patient at considerable risk of being injured by the seizure disorder itself. Even when a lapse in consciousness causes a fall, producing a head injury, the fall is often interpreted as the reason for the patient's confusion, and epilepsy is not suspected.

Of course, not all alterations of consciousness are the result of seizure activity. Any patient who is thought to have seizures should be investigated for other explanations as well. In the elderly, cardiac problems, such as subtle irregularities in the rhythm of the heart, can profoundly affect the flow of blood to the brain and produce transient unconsciousness. A Holter monitor recording of cardiac activity over the course of 24 hours may be needed to detect the irregular rhythm. Younger people may have metabolic or structural problems that cause fainting. In some, coughing or urinating will trigger an exaggerated vascular (vasovagal) reflex and induce fainting. Hyperventilation, an aberrant breathing pattern that commonly develops with acute anxiety, may also produce fainting and may be mistaken for a seizure disorder. Despite its popularity as a diagnosis, transient hypoglycemia rarely is responsible for fainting in people who are not taking medication to lower their blood sugar.[2]

History and Exam

With epilepsy, as with any medical complaint, the first step in the physician's investigation is to take a "history." This includes accounts by the patient, his family, and other witnesses of what happened during the seizure, during the days and weeks about the time of the seizure, and during other illnesses the patient may have had. Unfortunately, an accurate history is difficult to obtain in the case of epilepsy. The patient is often unaware of what occurred during the seizure and may have a confused and incomplete memory of events immediately preceding and following it. Family and friends are usually better sources for descriptions of the events surrounding the seizure, but they also may be too upset to remember exactly what happened. Since treatment is dictated by the type of seizure and the type of seizure is determined largely by the description of seizure characteristics, every attempt should be made to give the physician a complete and accurate picture of the seizure.

To complicate matters, many patients deliberately conceal

information relevant to their disorder. The patient may be too embarrassed to report bedwetting, and the family may fail to mention personality changes in the patient for fear of angering or offending him. If the seizures have evolved from fainting attacks to generalized convulsions, the patient and the family may cling to an early diagnosis of hypoglycemia or hardening of the arteries and not fully discuss the changing pattern of the attacks. Obviously, the evaluation of any patient with episodes suggestive of altered consciousness, transient involuntary movements, or fleeting sensory phenomena must include a series of questions that clarify what the patient has been experiencing. Urinary and fecal incontinence and tongue biting must be asked about specifically. Because aimless violence, personality changes, and sexual dysfunction are rarely recognized by the patient himself, other members of the family must be questioned pointedly about them. What happens during the seizure itself can be described only by witnesses, not by the patient.

A complete physical examination is basic to the investigation of every patient suspected of having a seizure disorder. Special attention to the nervous system is appropriate, but careful observation of all other major body systems is also important. Large brown spots over several areas of the skin may indicate neurofibromatosis, a hereditary disorder that can cause brain tumors. Minor joint changes may be the first indication of systemic lupus erythematosus, a vascular disease that can cause transient brain dysfunctions. A complete physical examination will also help to exclude problems that imitate seizures. An irregular pulse may be the first indication of an unsuspected cardiac arrhythmia. A heart murmur may prompt investigations that reveal valvular heart disease responsible for blood clots that periodically break off the diseased valves and go to the brain.

Electroencephalography

Most useful in the investigation of seizure disorders is the electroencephalograph, a device for amplifying and displaying changes in the electrical activity of the most superficial layers of the brain. Electrodes placed on the scalp detect fluctuations in voltage originating in several different areas of the brain. These fluctuations are amplified by special circuits in the electroencephalograph and are displayed as oscillations of voltage-sensitive needles. As the needles are deflected up and down with changes in the voltage, the pattern of changes is recorded on paper by ink released from the tips of the needles onto a constantly moving sheet of paper. This record of what are called brain waves is the electroencephalogram (EEG). In most cases, the electroencephalogram will help to establish the authenticity of the seizure disorder, and in some cases it can even suggest the underlying cause. Although an abnormal electroencephalogram can occur in someone who does not have seizures, it is good evidence that seizures are occurring in a patient with poorly understood motor, sensory, or psychic phenomena.

Several patterns of brain waves are normal in children and adults. When the patient is relaxed and has both eyes closed, rhythmical oscillations in electrical activity arising from the back part of the head will appear with a frequency of about eight to twelve cycles per second (hertz). This eight-to-twelve-hertz activity, called alpha activity, disappears when the patient opens his eyes or attempts intellectual tasks such as multiplication or division (see Figure 10.1). More toward the front of the head, the electroencephalogram will consist of irregular combinations of waves at varying frequencies. With drowsiness the overall frequency of the record slows.[3]

The electroencephalograph displays brain activity as waves, spikes, and electrical silence. A wave that is sharply contoured and lasts less than one-fifth of a second is called a sharp wave. When a sharply contoured wave lasts less than one-twelfth of a second, it is called a spike. Seizure activity usually appears as spikes or slow waves. Spikes and slow waves arising from a limited area over the brain generally indicate structural abnormalities in or near that part of the brain (Figure 10.2). There are several exceptions to this rule, and being aware of those exceptions keeps the physician from diagnosing brain disorders where they do not exist. Sharp waves, for example, may be normal at the back of the head in an elderly person. Spikes that appear to be pointing downward and occur at fourteen or six cycles per second, called fourteen- and six-per-second positive

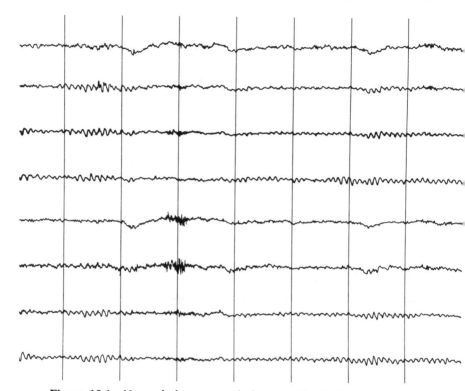

Figure 10.1 Normal electroencephalogram. The darker vertical lines on this record indicate 1-second intervals. The fourth and eighth horizontal lines most clearly show the small rhythmical waves called alpha waves. This young man had alpha waves with a frequency of 10 per second. The small spikes in the middle of the sixth and seventh horizontal lines are from muscle activity about the head.

spikes, usually appear to arise in the temporal regions in healthy young adults or adolescents. They may appear during sleep and do not indicate epilepsy. With arousal from sleep, there may be high-voltage wave activity with small notches that resemble spikes and slow waves. These are generally seen in childhood and are normal. All of these variants can lead to considerable misinterpretation of the electroencephalogram, especially when a seizure is suspected.[4]

Various maneuvers will make abnormal brain activity more apparent. Hyperventilation or sleep may enhance a spike focus

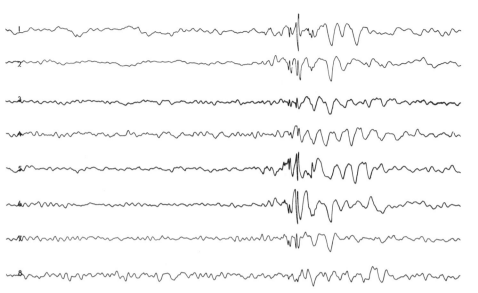

Figure 10.2 Spike-and-slow-wave discharge. Two-thirds of the way across the page there is a high-amplitude spike with associated high-amplitude slow waves. This type of activity often appears between seizures in a person with epilepsy. The areas most involved with the abnormal electrical activity are likely to be the regions of the brain in which the seizure activity is originating.

that is not prominent when the patient is awake or breathing at a normal rate. Flashing lights may elicit spike activity in an otherwise normal electroencephalogram. Spike activity arising on the mesial or inner surface of the temporal lobe may require special electrode arrangements for recording. One type of special electrode intended for this type of recording is the nasopharyngeal lead: this electrode is inserted into the nose and set against the lateral aspect of the nasopharynx so that it lies close to the inner face of the temporal lobe.

Although the electroencephalogram alone will not firmly establish the cause of the seizure disorder, some patterns limit the possible causes of the brain damage. Periodic discharges occurring at a rate of less than one discharge every four seconds often develop with subacute sclerosing panencephalitis, a rare but lethal degenerative disease of the brain. When the discharge rate is greater than once every two seconds, the underlying brain disease may be Creutzfeld-Jakob disease, a slow-viral illness causing dementia in adults, or Tay-Sachs disease, an inborn error of metabolism causing dementia in children. With brain disease resulting from poisons or anoxia, a periodic pattern occasionally appears in which wave activity is largely absent between discharges. This is called periodic lateralized epileptiform discharges, or PLEDS. Tumors, strokes, or other severe progressive lesions may produce PLEDS, and focal seizures often appear in patients with PLEDS.[5]

Other Tools for Diagnosing Epilepsy

The most useful diagnostic tool developed in the past decade is the computed tomogram (CT or CAT scan), a machine that transmits a fine beam of x-rays through the brain and uses a computer to interpret radiation absorption. The computer uses this information to create a picture of the brain as it would appear if it were sliced straight through at various angles. This machine has greatly simplified the identification of brain tumors, abscesses, and strokes. Equally promising computerized techniques are being developed to visualize both the structure and the metabolic activity of the brain. Nuclear magnetic resonance (NMR) provides a view of brain structure that should be even more revealing than computed tomography; it uses magnetic fields rather than ionizing radiation. Positron emission tomography (PET scanning) uses radioactive materials to reveal metabolic changes in the brain in very limited areas. It has been used in clinical studies, but it is still primarily a research tool. Because the radioactive isotopes needed for its operation are expensive and cumbersome to produce, it will probably see much less practical application than nuclear magnetic resonance. Strictly electrical approaches to the brain include evoked potential studies, which combine electroencephalographic techniques with computerized analysis of minute changes in brain activity. All of these recently developed techniques have made the evaluation of individuals with epilepsy much simpler and more accurate.[6]

More conventional techniques also provide information on the origin of seizures. Studies of the blood and spinal fluid are usually helpful in eliminating several possible causes of nervous system disease. In systemic lupus erythematosus, abnormal antibodies are apparent in the blood, and in bacterial meningitis the responsible organism is usually found in the spinal fluid. When blood vessel abnormalities are suspected, angiography is used to visualize the intracranial vessels. Until a few years ago, a catheter to inject radiographic dye had to be introduced directly into the major arteries to the head, a procedure involving small but real risks. With the computerized system called digital subtraction angiography, the dye can be injected into a vein in a limb and still be used to visualize the intracranial arteries. Manipulation of a vein is less risky than threading a catheter through an artery. Digital subtraction angiography has the additional advantage of requiring little skill on the part of the individual introducing the dye.

Origin of Seizures

As we have already seen, seizure disorders may develop from obvious central nervous system disease (symptomatic epilepsy) or independently of any apparent nervous system defect (idiopathic epilepsy). Particular causes of the disorder, when they can be identified, are more or less likely depending on the age of the patient. Some causes of epilepsy are specific for a particular age (see Chapter 6). In newborns, birth asphyxia and hereditary metabolic problems are often responsible for seizures, whereas in children, head injuries and nervous system infections are more likely to be the cause. The middle-aged adult developing seizures for the first time often has a brain tumor or a vascular problem (Box 10.1). Seizures at any age that are initially well controlled and later recur despite antiepileptic drugs may arise from structural brain damage: tumors, abscesses, or blood clots in or over the brain; inflammatory disorders or malformations of the blood vessels to the brain; or congenital defects in the formation of the brain.[7]

Signs and symptoms associated with the seizure disorder are often helpful in determining its precise cause. Metabolic problems are usually accompanied by impaired thinking or coordination. A rapidly progressive paralysis or speech disorder associated with an obvious infection in the ear suggests a brain abscess extending from the disease in the ear. People with abnormal pigmentation in the skin or obvious vascular abnormalities over the face (port-wine nevi) are at high risk of having associated nervous system tumors.[8]

Idiopathic Epilepsy

Most generalized absence (petit mal) seizures and the majority of complex partial (psychomotor) seizures develop for no apparent reason. Generalized tonic-clonic (grand mal) seizures may appear after major head trauma or a central nervous system infection, but more often they too develop without any obvious cause. In many cases, examination of the brain at autopsy of someone who had epilepsy all his life will reveal no abnormalities that could account for the seizure disorder. People whose seizures are not explained by structural damage to the brain or metabolic defects in the nervous system are assumed to have subtle problems at the level of interactions between small areas of the brain or individual nerve cells. Much of the brain's activity is inhibitory, and so it is likely that impaired function in one part of the brain can allow abnormal activity, such as seizures, to develop in another part of the brain.[9]

The idea that damage to the brain occurs before or at birth in patients with idiopathic seizures has been popular for several decades, but it is difficult to prove. The common fear that a child delivered with the assistance of forceps would suffer brain damage and develop epilepsy is baseless. In fact, during a difficult birth, properly applied forceps can provide additional protection to the newborn's head and can reduce pressure against the skull as the child leaves the birth canal. Whether temporary oxygen deprivation to the brain during birth plays a role in idiopathic seizures is still controversial.

Posttraumatic Seizures

Head injuries can cause substantial brain damage and are a common cause of seizures in both children and adults. Any adult in whom head trauma leads to focal neurologic deficits, such as paralysis of an arm, loss of vision in one visual field, or loss of sensation over one side of the body, is at very high risk of developing seizures, but seizures can occur days or months after a serious head injury even when there are no signs of permanent brain damage (Figure 10.3). If there is a skull fracture, prolonged loss of consciousness, or obvious brain damage associated with the trauma, seizures are likely to appear as a delayed effect of the injury. Seizures occurring at the time of an injury, called impact seizures, are an indication that the head trauma is severe. If focal damage occurs in the brain, such as a blood clot in the temporal lobe, the patient often develops partial seizures.[10]

When the injury to the brain is slight and no obvious tissue damage has occurred, the injury is called a concussion. People who have had concussions usually complain of headache, may have some temporary difficulty with memory, and often have lingering dizziness and sleep disorders. Epilepsy should not develop after a concussion. With more serious injury, the brain

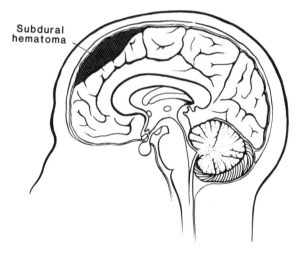

Subdural
hematoma

Figure 10.3 Subdural hematoma. Relatively minor trauma in elderly people can produce blood clots that overlie the brain and may produce signs of brain damage. An elderly person with confusion, weakness, and seizures may be thought to have had a stroke, but the actual problem may be a head injury that caused bleeding inside the skull.

may be bruised and swell from the pooling of tissue fluids and blood. In this type of injury, called a contusion, the risk of later developing a seizure disorder is substantial. A contusion can occur even when the skull is not fractured, but trauma sufficient to produce a contusion often fractures the skull. The victim of the trauma will usually lose consciousness for more than five minutes after the impact. Memory of the episode and even of events immediately preceding the episode will be defective. Weakness in a limb, speech problems, double vision, vertigo, and changes in sensitivity to pain may occur. The extent to which these focal neurologic deficits will resolve will depend upon the size and location of the contusion. Focal motor or focal sensory seizures may appear long after the patient recovers from massive head trauma.

Postinfectious Seizures

An infection of the brain itself is called encephalitis; an infection primarily affecting the lining around the brain and spinal cord is called meningitis. Meningitis and encephalitis frequently cause seizures when they are active, and even after the infection clears up the patient faces substantial risk of developing a seizure disorder. Early in the course of the infection, a viral or bacterial encephalitis may produce a confusing picture of altered behavior, movement disorders, and partial or generalized seizures, but within days or weeks of these symptoms the more serious character of the disease is usually apparent. Fever, neck stiffness, and progressive impairment of consciousness routinely develop with the infection. The organism responsible for the infection is less important than the severity of the infection in determining the likelihood that epilepsy will develop after the patient has recovered. Seizures that develop after nervous system infections are usually generalized.[11]

Parasitic Disease

Parasites that invade the brain or deposit eggs in the brain account for a large proportion of seizure disorders in some countries. Cysticercosis from the pork tapeworm *Taenia solium* is especially common in Mexico and is often seen in the Philippines. Schistosomiasis is widespread in the less industrialized areas of the Orient, and cerebral malaria is still a frequent cause of acute seizure disorders in tropical countries. Although the parasite may not cause much damage through its own activity in the nervous system, the nervous system's reaction to the foreign agent may produce a "scar" that serves as the focus for the seizure activity. Control of seizures in individuals with parasitic disease of the nervous system does not depend upon eradication of the parasite. Complete seizure control can be achieved even when structural damage to the brain from the parasite is obvious. The seizures that do develop may be partial or generalized.

Tumor-Related Seizures

Seizures that appear in an adult who has had no history of childhood or adolescent seizures, has suffered no trauma, is not alcoholic, has not had a stroke, and does not have an infection of the central nervous system are commonly caused by a tumor in the brain. These qualifications make this cause of seizures relatively infrequent simply because trauma, alcoholism, stroke, and infection are common in adults. Brain tumors are seldom the cause of seizures in childhood, because tumors in children are usually at the base of the brain in the brainstem and the cerebellum, areas of injury that usually do not provoke a seizure disorder.

With most tumors, the patient will have focal weakness, sensory loss, or psychological changes associated with the seizures, but even when none of these other signs is present the tumor may be highly invasive. If the tumor cannot be cured, control of the seizures with anticonvulsants may fail as the tumor extends. Seizures that develop with tumors may be partial or generalized, but they will usually reflect the part of the brain most damaged by the growth. For example, an occipital lobe tumor may cause visual hallucinations, whereas a frontal lobe tumor may produce twitching in an arm or a leg.

Box 10.1
Causes of Epilepsy in Adults

Idiopathic

Trauma

Infection

Stroke

Hemorrhage

Tumor

Vascular malformation

Vascular inflammation

Parasites

Poisons

Drugs

Vascular Disease

A variety of transient and permanent blood vessel disorders may produce seizures as the first sign of disease or may allow seizures to develop long after they have done considerable damage in the nervous system and elsewhere. A common disease that occasionally causes epilepsy is stroke. A relatively uncommon vascular disease that frequently causes seizures is systemic lupus erythematosus. The type of person affected and the problems associated with the epilepsy vary with the vascular disorder.

Stroke. A stroke is damage to the brain caused by inadequate blood flow. That damage may occur because a blood vessel is obstructed by cholesterol collecting in the wall of the vessel (atherosclerosis) or because a weakened vessel bursts and bleeds into the brain. In patients with diseased heart valves, small blood clots may form on the rough surfaces of the damaged valves and then travel to the head and obstruct blood flow in the brain. Structural damage late in life from stroke or from a transient drop in the level of blood oxygen (hypoxia) may lead to generalized or partial seizures within weeks or months. Epilepsy occasionally develops years after a stroke. If it appears after a delay of months or years, the old stroke cannot be held responsible until other possible causes, such as a metastatic tumor or a meningitis, are eliminated. Even when the stroke occurs shortly before the onset of seizures, it cannot simply be assumed to be the cause of the seizure disorder. Other problems must be looked for. If none is found, the stroke should be considered the cause of the epilepsy.[12]

Vascular malformation. Abnormal networks of blood vessels develop in the brains of some people while the nervous system is still forming, but the vascular malformation often remains inapparent until adulthood. Although the first indication of a malformation may be a lethal hemorrhage from the primitive blood vessels, changes associated with these vascular lesions are often more subtle. Vascular malformations in the brain cause changes in the pattern of blood flow that can lead to seizures even when the malformation is small. Seizures are also caused by vascular malformations that produce small hemorrhages in the brain or simply grow into a large mass in the head.

Vasculitis. Any inflammation of blood vessels is called vasculitis. Some types of vasculitis arise from infection, some from allergic reactions, and some are idiopathic. An occasional cause of generalized or complex partial seizures in young adults is systemic lupus erythematosus, an inflammatory disease that can affect the blood vessels in the brain, as well as elsewhere, and decrease blood flow to large areas of the brain. The central nervous system is damaged (but often reversibly) in 59 percent of patients with lupus. Of these, 17 to 50 percent will have seizures. Psychiatric problems are also commonly associated with this inflammatory disease, and many patients with seizures caused by lupus will have depression or other changes in mood that confuse the diagnostic picture.[13]

Metabolic Disorders

Profoundly abnormal changes in the levels of calcium, sodium, and glucose in the blood may be responsible for generalized tonic-clonic seizures in otherwise normal people. Elevated blood urea nitrogen from kidney failure and other toxic products from liver failure can also evoke seizures. When the patient has abnormal blood chemistry, there are invariably other clinical signs of the metabolic problem, but they may be obscured by the seizures. Chronic metabolic disorders from hereditary metabolic diseases are less common, but they too are occasionally responsible for epilepsy. Some, like Tay-Sachs disease, are frequently checked for in newborns.[14]

Poisoning, another type of metabolic derangement, may also cause seizures. Children are particularly likely to develop generalized seizures with nervous system damage from lead poisoning. Thallium, a poison that resembles salt, and carbon monoxide, an odorless gas occasionally emitted by faulty heating systems as well as by automobiles, may cause brain damage that induces seizures at any age. Poisoning is often difficult to detect, and so a patient may suffer from generalized seizures for weeks or months before other signs suggest poison as the cause of the epilepsy.

Seizures Related to Alcohol and Drugs

Partial and generalized seizures often develop in alcoholics because of head injuries that occur during the period of intoxication or because of withdrawal from the alcohol. Alcohol withdrawal seizures, also known as rum fits, can occur after as little as 24 hours of alcohol abuse. They occur in 4 percent of patients who go on to develop delirium tremens, the acute thought disorder that affects some chronic alcoholics who are denied alcohol for a few days.[15]

Seizure disorders related to alcohol abuse most commonly appear after adolescence, and they are always a diagnostic and therapeutic problem. The diagnostic difficulty arises because people who are intoxicated are especially likely to have had head injuries, and so even a patient who appears several times a year with rum fits must be evaluated for a variety of brain injuries including cerebral contusions, subdural hematomas, and post-traumatic meningitis. The therapeutic difficulties arise from the behavioral and biochemical characteristics of the chronic alcoholic. Drug compliance is erratic when these patients are not intoxicated and breaks down entirely when they are intoxicated. Even if the medication is given on a regular basis by a friend or family member, the rate of breakdown and excretion of antiepileptic drugs is altered by chronic drinking. Phenytoin, for example, is turned over more quickly in an alcoholic without terminal liver damage than in a normal person or in an alcoholic with advanced cirrhosis of the liver.

Although status epilepticus—a series of closely spaced seizures—often occurs with drug withdrawal, alcoholics show no exaggerated risk of developing it. To some extent alcohol acts as an antiepileptic; seizures occur when the level of alcohol falls. This does not mean a person cannot have seizures while drunk. In fact, seizures often occur while alcoholics are still very intoxicated. Presumably, shifting levels of alcohol in the brain and brain damage associated with the alcoholism work together to provoke seizures.

A variety of other agents that are commonly used illicitly or with medical supervision can evoke seizures in susceptible individuals. Antidepressants, stimulants, antipsychotic medications, and sleep preparations all occasionally allow seizures. With some medications, such as barbiturates in sleep preparations, the seizures appear when the medication is discontinued. Tricyclic antidepressants, such as imipramine (Tofranil) and amitriptyline (Elavil), presumably lower the seizure threshold directly and increase the risk of seizure activity as the blood level of the drug rises.

The effects of other illicit substances on seizure frequency are controversial. Despite the widespread use of marijuana, cocaine, amphetamines, and methaqualone (Quaalude) as recreational drugs in the United States, little objective study of their contribution to the incidence and control of seizure disorders has been possible. Aside from restrictions on the use of the drugs for scientific studies, a major complicating factor has been the misrepresentation of the drugs that people actually obtain through illegal sources. Much of what is sold as cocaine is adulterated, and these unpredictable impurities are likely to be as active as the illicit drug in the mixture.

One patient whose seizures had been well controlled for more than a year despite occasional cocaine use developed a complex partial seizure a few days after using material given to her as a present and alleged to be high-quality cocaine. She suspected that the drug was adulterated because it seemed less potent than cocaine she had used in the past. She guessed that the cocaine had been mixed with an amphetamine, because it caused mood changes similar to ones she had had in the past when taking amphetamines. That her seizure occurred while she was on phenytoin and shortly after she used the illicit drug implicated the illicit drug as a contributing factor. But what she had actually inhaled could not be determined. The same problems of adulteration occur with all illicit drugs. For this reason even if for no other, illegal drugs present special problems for people with epilepsy and should be avoided.

Pseudoseizures

People who do not have epilepsy, and even some who do, occasionally pretend to have seizures. These pseudoseizures or factitious seizures are most often contrived to gain attention and sympathy or to avoid responsibilities. Contrived seizures would have little effect if they could be recognized for what they are, but determining whether a seizure is authentic or not is difficult, even when the observer is familiar with epilepsy. Even experienced neurologists can identify factitious seizures in only three out of four instances.[16]

Factitious seizures occur in both children and adults. Women have them somewhat more often than men, but they are common in both sexes. They usually begin between the ages of 22 and 32. People with pseudoseizures have a much higher than average incidence of psychiatric disease, including depressive illnesses and suicide attempts, in their families. Individuals with contrived seizures also often have obvious sexual problems, such as impotence or exhibitionism. Although pseudoseizures are routinely called hysterical seizures or conversion reactions, terms that suggest an emotional or thought disorder, they are not necessarily caused by a psychiatric problem. They are primarily a learned response to situations and responsibilities, a technique that abruptly shifts control into the hands of the person having the attack. They can be a powerful tool with which to manipulate family, friends, and unsuspecting strangers.

Pseudoseizures have their disadvantages as well. The person who has them is unnecessarily exposed to the risks of diagnostic tests, as well as to the side effects of anticonvulsants on the blood, liver, kidneys, and nervous system. Diane, the young wife of a busy and successful executive, had increasingly frequent generalized convulsions that resisted all anticonvulsant therapy. She and her husband agreed to highly invasive studies of the brain and surgery on the brain if necessary as a last effort to control the seizures. On the transcontinental flight to the diagnostic center where the surgery was to be performed, she had seizures that abated only with massive doses of intravenous medication. Her husband was constantly at her side throughout the ordeal. Extensive testing at the diagnostic center revealed no true seizure activity. Diane's pseudoseizures gained her an extraordinary amount of attention from her family and physicians, but at a less careful institution she would have faced procedures that posed considerable risks for her. Even if she had ultimately refused surgery, the diagnostic studies justified by the apparently life-threatening severity of her seizure disorder would have exposed her to risks that were unjustifiable in the assessment of what proved to be a psychiatric problem.

If the family realizes the attacks are contrived, the person who has developed pseudoseizures to avoid conflict may find himself even more deeply embroiled in conflict. The patient's seizures may become more severe as the family tries to discredit the epilepsy as a real problem. If the family does not know that the seizures are contrived, considerable time and effort may be spent in a futile attempt to suppress them.

Clinical Features of Pseudoseizures

No one without epilepsy should be exposed to the risks of anticonvulsant medication, and anyone who contrives fits to make life simpler needs psychiatric help to develop less destructive techniques for dealing with friends and family. Since most people with pseudoseizures are not medically sophisticated, their seizures often display characteristics that make their authenticity questionable. But before abandoning attempts to control the seizures with medication, the physician must be very sure the episodes are contrived. Establishing this is often quite difficult even with the help of monitors of brain electrical activity. However, there are some reliable principles to follow in determining whether seizures are authentic.

Factitious seizures, like true seizures, have characteristics that appear repeatedly. In each person with pseudoseizures, the same symptoms and behavior occur in the same sequence with each episode. The pattern that pseudoseizures assume varies somewhat with different cultures and historical periods, but the similarity is more striking than the variability. During the nineteenth century, animal-like movements were common; currently the most common type of pseudoseizure involves limb movements. Three out of four patients with pseudoseizures make no response or bizarre responses to verbal stimuli during their fits. Over 80 percent have abnormal movements, and 70 percent complain of nausea, cramps, abdominal pain, bad tastes, or other symptoms related to the mouth or gastrointestinal tract. About one-third have an apparent change in their breathing patterns, and nearly half speak, grunt, moan, sob, cough, hum, or make other types of nonverbal noises during the attack.

Semipurposeful behavior is evident in more than half of patients having a pseudoseizure. Complaints before, during, or after the factitious seizure routinely include dizziness, head pain, visual changes, feelings of depersonalization, hot flashes, auditory changes, and other less easily described total-body changes. The most common motor phenomena include grimacing, posturing of the limbs or trunk, trembling, limb jerking, and limb flailing. Violent behavior is rare, but the patient may run, cry, make obscene gestures, or chew purposelessly. Choking, gagging, lip smacking or licking, and hyperventilation are common. This abnormal behavior usually lasts longer than similar phenomena occurring in true seizures.

A pseudoseizure is difficult to distinguish from a complex partial (psychomotor) seizure unless the patient is attached to an electroencephalograph at the time of the episode. More helpful than what happens during the seizure is what happens after it. As in many authentic complex partial seizures, the patient's abnormal movements may include or progress to tonic-clonic limb and body movements, but unlike the victim of an authentic seizure, the unsophisticated patient with pseudoseizures may respond purposefully and talk within seconds of the tonic-clonic phase of a lengthy pseudoseizure. There is no postictal phase with cessation of the movements. The patient may open his eyes and report, "I had a fit," or simply look around with surprise and ask, "What was that?" Patients rarely suffer injuries during contrived fits, and only the most sophisticated patients will urinate during these episodes. Most will resist any efforts to interfere with their breathing during the ictal phase. This contrasts dramatically with the severe difficulty in breathing that some patients suffer during true seizures without making any effort to clear the airway.

Epilepsy and Pseudoseizures

Patients who have had true seizures for several years are best able to contrive seizures, but these are precisely the patients who must be assumed to be having true seizures until evidence of pseudoseizures is overwhelming. Of patients with intractable seizures, 8 to 20 percent have both pseudoseizures and true seizures. Factitious seizures occur in patients with all types of epileptic disorders. A history of psychological problems is often lacking, and the people involved with the patient are therefore obliged to assume the seizures are authentic. Any secondary gain provided by the pseudoseizures is usually fairly obvious, but the fact that the patient gains something from the seizure activity does not prove that the seizures are contrived.

If all of a patient's attacks are contrived, an electroencephalogram obtained during a seizure will usually indicate that it is factitious. The record will be normal except for the electrical activity generated by muscle activity as the patient moves about. But obtaining such a recording to rule out true seizures may be impossible with a sophisticated patient. One way to make pseudoseizures easier to detect is to use tape recording equipment that goes everywhere with the patient. Continuous monitoring of the patient, especially if combined with videotaping, makes it possible to observe and analyze several episodes. By studying these recurrent episodes, the physician can usually tell whether they are authentic.

Detecting pseudoseizures in a patient who also has true seizures is more difficult. About 90 percent of patients with epilepsy show abnormal brain waves on the electroencephalogram during the interval between true seizures (the interictal period). Therefore an abnormal electroencephalogram is often seen during or shortly after a pseudoseizure, and this makes diagnosis difficult in these patients. But several *normal* records obtained shortly after seizures are highly suggestive of a contrived seizure disorder.

Family Members with Imitated Seizures

Contrived seizures occasionally appear in relatives of a person with epilepsy. In fact, family members who have witnessed the authentic seizures may imitate them very convincingly. Children are especially likely to reenact the seizure activity they observe in their parents or siblings. Factitious epilepsy becomes a game for some children, or a way of getting their share of attention. Adults rarely imitate the seizures exhibited by one of their children. Because close relatives of a person with epilepsy are at higher risk of developing seizures than the general population, any seizures in siblings or children of people with epilepsy must be considered authentic until evidence to the contrary is overwhelming.

Chapter 11

Treatment

There are several types of treatment for epilepsy. What therapy is most appropriate depends primarily upon the type of epilepsy the patient has. Antiepileptic drugs are usually given before other therapies are tried, and most patients will be free of seizures while they are taking appropriate drugs. As I have emphasized throughout this book, being free of seizures means having the opportunity to lead a relatively normal life. Incomplete control that develops after a long seizure-free period can often be traced to changes in the patient's lifestyle, general health, or level of compliance. Adjusting the dose or scheduling of drugs once serum drug levels have been checked will usually ensure a return to good seizure control.

Unfortunately, some people have persistently poor seizure control despite appropriate modifications in their lifestyles, medication regimens, and cooperation. For a few, recurrent or refractory seizures are a sign of new or extended disease of the central nervous system. For others, the intractable seizure activity has no treatable basis and provides a constant source of frustration and despair.

No case of intractable seizures should be considered hopeless just because currently available treatments are ineffective; new drugs are being tested and introduced every year. This search for better drugs continues even though antiepileptic medications now available can eliminate or decrease the frequency of most types of seizures. Researchers continue to seek drugs that can be taken infrequently and that suppress the seizures without causing adverse reactions. Side effects limit the usefulness of all of the antiepileptic drugs now available: allergic reactions, gastrointestinal distress, lethargy, impotence, or confusion make some patients unable to take the medication that is most effective against their type of seizure disorder. Fortunately, with most of the drugs used, the side effects are relatively minor, considering the independence and security they provide.

For people with seizures that do not respond to conventional medications, alternative treatments include surgery and dietary approaches. But regardless of what type of treatment the person with epilepsy receives, getting involved with other patients with similar problems is usually helpful. Meetings of similarly affected families can reduce frustrations, especially when seizure control is poor, by providing new perspectives and strategies. Patients are often more frank with other patients than with their physician. They do not want to alienate the physician, because they may need him in the future, but in talking to other patients and families there is no reason to gloss over medication lapses or eccentric therapies.

Effectiveness of Treatment

Most people with epilepsy have fewer or less severe seizures when they take antiepileptic medication. How well an individual will respond to drugs is affected by several factors, including the type of central nervous system problem causing the epilepsy, nonneurologic problems associated with the epilepsy, and the patient's ability to absorb and metabolize the drug. Despite these many variables, the likelihood that a particular patient will do well on medication is fairly predictable.

The patients who respond best to drugs are those with idiopathic epilepsy, that is, those with no apparent explanation for their seizure disorders (see Box 11.1). Even when there is an obvious basis for the seizure disorder, such as an old head injury or meningitis, the less frequent the seizure episodes, the better the level of control that can be achieved. The patient's age also affects the likelihood of complete seizure control with medication: seizures that appear before age 10 are generally more easily controlled than those appearing later, but if seizures appear in the child's first year the outlook is poor. (This excludes simple febrile seizures, a problem common in infants and not indicative of long-term epilepsy.) The poor outcome when seizures appear before one year of age is probably due to the high probability of congenital brain damage in this group of patients. An especially worrisome sign is the association of a profoundly abnormal electroencephalogram (hypsarrhythmia) with associated body and limb jerks (infantile spasms) in an infant. Infants with

---

Box 11.1
Outlook for Complete Seizure Control

Good	*Poor*
Strictly generalized seizures	Complex partial seizures with tonic-clonic activity as well
Strictly complex partial seizures	
Idiopathic basis for seizures	Seizures from tumor, stroke, contusion, meningitis, etc.
No intellectual impairment	Low I.Q.
No personality disorder	Obvious personality disorder
Normal EEG or minor background abnormalities	Anterior temporal or frontal lobe abnormalities on EEG
Treatment begun within 1 year of seizure onset	Treatment delayed
Onset at 2 to 5 years of age	Onset before 1 year of age

hypsarrhythmia may develop brain damage if treatment of seizures is delayed even a few days, but even with early treatment, the outlook for seizure control and relatively normal intellectual development in these children is poor.[1]

Good seizure control is most easily achieved in patients who start taking antiepileptic drugs within a year of their first seizure. Epilepsy is more likely to be fully controlled if it is treated early and aggressively than if it is allowed to recur in the hope that the patient will grow out of it without treatment.

Seizure control is more elusive if the patient has more than one type of seizure, a grossly abnormal neurologic examination, a low IQ score, or a severe personality disorder. Electrical studies of the brain can sometimes help detect patients who are likely to respond poorly to antiepileptic medication, but the patient's history is usually more useful than any specific pattern on the electroencephalogram. If a discrete event caused the seizure disorder, the type of event will correlate with the probability of seizure control. Epilepsy that develops after a massive head injury is not likely to remit completely on any anticonvulsant regimen, whereas people whose seizures are caused by strokes or central nervous system infections usually achieve good control with a single anticonvulsant. Probably the most important factor in determining the level of seizure control is the type of seizure disorder the patient has.

Of patients who remain free of seizures during their first year of treatment, 87 percent will have no seizures for at least three years if they continue the treatment. With appropriate anticonvulsant therapy, complete elimination of seizures is possible in about 60 percent of people with partial seizures. This relatively high level of control occurs in individuals with both simple (focal motor; focal sensory) and some types of complex partial seizures. With generalized tonic-clonic (grand mal) epilepsy, complete control of seizures is feasible in 69 percent of people treated with the best drugs currently available. This is about the same level of control that can be achieved in generalized absence (petit mal) seizures. Taking all seizure types together, only about 9 percent of patients on standard anticonvulsant treatment show no response to the drugs, and at least 58 percent have complete seizure control.

The electroencephalogram may remain distinctly abnormal even while the patient is seizure-free. Improvement in seizure control usually precedes electroencephalographic improvement. A persistently abnormal electroencephalogram years after the seizures begin is not a sign of future seizure activity, even though such abnormal brain wave patterns early after the first seizure often do predict more seizure activity. Anticonvulsant drugs may return the patient to a normal level of functioning even though the brain has obvious electrical abnormalities.

Follow-up by Physicians

The more closely patients are followed by physicians, the better their seizure control usually is. Patients who are willing to see a doctor are often also willing to comply with the doctor's instructions. When seizure control is poor, the patient is more likely to be skeptical of the treatment and to experiment with unorthodox therapies. Despite the reluctance of those most in need of supervision—those with poor seizure control—to submit to it, a substantial improvement in control can often be achieved if the physician makes a concerted effort to monitor the patient directly or with the cooperation of the family.

During a patient's first year of taking an antiepileptic drug, several follow-up visits to the physician are essential. Within a few weeks of starting the medication, blood tests will show if the patient is tolerating the medication and if enough of it is getting into the bloodstream. If seizure control is poor or side effects of the medication are a problem, the patient may need a change in the dose or the type of drug used. During these visits, the physician also has an opportunity to see if any new information about the cause of the seizure disorder has surfaced. The physician can also reinforce instructions on taking the medication and answer the patient's or family's questions under circumstances that are less stressful than those of the first visit.

When seizure control is complete, follow-up examinations by a doctor familiar with the problem may be necessary only once a year. If any dramatic changes in health or lifestyle occur, however, the physician should be consulted to see if any adjustments in antiepileptic medication will be needed.

Antiepileptic Drugs

Phenobarbital was introduced in 1912 and provided dramatic relief from seizures for many patients. Its inability to suppress all seizure types and its side effects, such as sedation in adults and hyperactivity in children, prompted the development of other anticonvulsants. Bromide salts were an early treatment that caused the sedation characteristic of phenobarbital and had the added disadvantage of causing acne, but seizure control was claimed for three out of four patients treated with bromides. However, the duration of the "complete" control has been ambiguously defined in many reports on the experience with particular anticonvulsants.[2]

Because the acceptability and long-term benefits of both phenobarbital and bromides were limited, other drugs were sought. Phenytoin entered clinical neurology in 1938 and immediately became the standard by which all other antiepileptics were measured. Most of the anticonvulsants developed had chemical ties to phenobarbital and phenytoin. Primidone was so closely related to phenobarbital that when it was first introduced there was controversy over whether its only active metabolite was phenobarbital. Ethosuximide and methsuximide had no advantages over phenytoin in most seizure disorders, but they proved more effective than other drugs in suppressing generalized absence (petit mal) seizures. Valproic acid is one of the few antiepileptic drugs with no structural similarity to phenobarbital or phenytoin. It has proved valuable in treating generalized seizure disorders, but it has disadvantages, such as liver toxicity, that have only recently become apparent.

For every anticonvulsant there is a therapeutic range—a concentration of drug in the blood that causes few or no side effects and gives maximum benefit to most patients who are sensitive to the drug. How much medication will produce a therapeutic level varies from person to person. Because of this, levels of the drug in the blood serum should be routinely checked in any patient responding poorly to a conventional dose of anticonvulsant medication.

All of the currently used antiepileptic drugs have adverse side effects. Most of the risks are the same for all patients taking a given medication, but there are noteworthy exceptions. Women trying to become pregnant while taking anticonvulsants must face the risk of birth defects (see Chapter 5). Some men may find that certain drugs, such as phenobarbital, make them impotent. Patients with chronic liver disease or alcoholism may not be able to tolerate drugs metabolized in the liver. The risk of un-wanted side effects is minimized by using the anticonvulsants that are most effective against the patient's seizure type (Box 11.2). Ideally, the seizures should be managed with only one antiepileptic drug, but some patients are not seizure-free on only one anticonvulsant. Two or three drugs in combination must be used in these refractory cases, and the likelihood of unwanted side effects is correspondingly increased.

Phenytoin

Phenytoin (Dilantin, Epanutin) is an effective anticonvulsant for some partial seizure disorders and is the drug of choice for gen-eralized tonic-clonic (grand mal) seizures. It is supplied as a

---

Box 11.2
Drugs of Choice According to
Type of Epilepsy

Seizure type	Anticonvulsant
Generalized tonic-clonic (grand mal)	Phenytoin
Complex partial (psycho-motor)	Carbamazepine
Generalized absence (petit mal)	Ethosuximide
Simple partial	Phenytoin

capsule, tablet, or syrup and is usually given in one or more doses daily. The average adult dose required to produce a therapeutic level of the drug in the blood is 300 milligrams (3 pills) daily. The therapeutic level is 10 to 20 micrograms per milliliter of serum.[3]

Although phenytoin occasionally produces blood disorders and allergic reactions, the more common serious reactions are nerologic and psychologic. A staggering gait, slurred speech, blurred vision, and mild sedation are the most frequent complaints, though many patients experience none of these side effects. On examination, the patient will have difficulty walking, abnormal eye movements, and mildly slurred speech as the serum level of the drug enters the toxic range. Some patients complain that the drug gives them an upset stomach or altered bowel patterns, but these problems are usually mild and transient. Decades of phenytoin use often cause persistent, but mild, gait problems and sensory loss. These result from injury to peripheral nerves and nervous system centers for balance control. The most disturbing side effect of phenytoin is its cosmetic effect. Women in particular complain of coarsening of facial features and darkening of limb and facial hair. Both men and women are often plagued by an overgrowth of the gums (gingival hyperplasia) that is unsightly and can lead to tooth loss.

Psychologic problems rarely occur as adverse reactions to phenytoin, but the range of psychologic reactions that do occur is broad. Many patients complain of intellectual slowing and poor concentration, and a very few patients have hallucinations. Confusion and disorientation are especially common in people who had minor problems in memory or thinking before taking the medication. The patient may report difficulty with memory or calculations, and family or friends may find the patient irascible. These complications may actually be caused by other drugs taken simultaneously that interfere with the breakdown of phenytoin. Drugs that commonly interfere with the metabolism of phenytoin include diazepam (Valium), chlorpromazine (Thorazine), prochlorperazine (Compazine), methylphenidate (Ritalin), cimetidine (Tagamet), and chlordiazepoxide (Librium).

If a patient develops a rash shortly after starting to take phenytoin, an allergy to the drug is assumed to be responsible and the drug will be stopped. Many patients develop new complaints, such as blurred vision or tremors, that may be from too high a level of phenytoin in the blood or from a problem unrelated to phenytoin. The simplest way to check for phenytoin toxicity is to obtain a blood serum level. The level of phenytoin in the serum should reach a plateau after the patient has been on the drug for about five days. With serum levels higher than 20 micrograms per milliliter, toxic signs and even increased seizure frequency may appear. Toxic effects aside from an acute allergic or gastrointestinal reaction should not arise for several hours after oral administration of the drug, because absorption is so slow that peak serum levels are not reached until about four to eight hours after an oral dose.

Attempts to commit suicide by taking an overdose of phenytoin are usually unsuccessful, because gastric irritation will trigger vomiting of a massive oral dose. Most patients find it difficult to take more than 500 milligrams (five capsules) at one time. If more than ten or fifteen capsules are swallowed and retained, the principal danger of the drug is in its cardiac action, though fatal arrhythmias rarely occur even after such massive oral doses. A rapid intravenous infusion of phenytoin carries substantial danger, but most patients do not have the means to inject the medication directly into the bloodstream, and phenytoin injected into muscle is very poorly absorbed.

Phenobarbital

Phenobarbital, one of the oldest anticonvulsants in use, is currently not the first choice for any type of seizure in adults. However, many pediatricians prefer it for several types of generalized and partial seizures because of its established safety and effectiveness in children. It is the drug of choice for treating complex febrile seizures in children. In adults with generalized seizure disorders, it is occasionally used as a second drug if the patient has persistent seizures while taking the drug of choice alone. The oral dose required to produce an anticonvulsant effect in adults ranges from about 90 to 200 milligrams (Box 11.3). The dose for children must be based on the age and size of the child. Phenobarbital is supplied as either a tablet or a syrup.[4]

Its high incidence of side effects has increasingly curtailed the use of phenobarbital as alternative drugs have been developed. Children given the drug sometimes become hyperactive, irritable, aggressive, and tearful. These hyperactive children have reduced attention spans, are easily distracted, and are destructive. Most adults have no adverse reactions to phenobarbital, except for mild sedation, until toxic levels are reached, and then they usually have a staggering gait, slurred speech, and abnormal eye movements. Marked confusion may develop in adults with serum phenobarbital levels of over 60 micrograms per milliliter, but this is so much in excess of the therapeutic range of 15 to 35 micrograms per milliliter that the patient will usually develop other signs first. Although the side effects of phenobarbital in young adults are relatively minor, several other antiepileptic drugs are more effective for specific seizure types at doses that produce less sedation. Elderly adults are more vulnerable to side effects of phenobarbital and may have restlessness, confusion, and severe depression at relatively low doses. Abrupt

---

Box 11.3
Therapeutic Levels

Drug	*Serum level**	*Oral adult dose***
Phenytoin	10–20	300–400
Carbamazepine	6–10	600–1200
Valproic acid	50–100	1000–3000
Ethosuximide	50–100	750–2000
Primidone	6–12	750–1500
Phenobarbital	15–35	120–250

*In micrograms of drug per milliliter of serum.
**Daily dose in milligrams usually needed to achieve therapeutic level.

withdrawal from phenobarbital may cause seizures even in patients with no previous seizures. Individuals at risk for this type of withdrawal seizure are those using phenobarbital for sedation or as a recreational drug.

The relatively high incidence of side effects with phenobarbital contributes to a high level of noncompliance in adult patients. About 20 percent of patients for whom it is prescribed do not take it as instructed or do not take it at all.

An additional disadvantage of phenobarbital is its potential for abuse. Patients may use the drug for its mood-altering effects or take an overdose in a suicide attempt. It is well tolerated orally, and the peak serum level is not reached until twelve to eighteen hours after an oral dose. An extremely high dose, many times more than would normally be prescribed, or the combination of phenobarbital with alcohol or other drugs may depress breathing and result in death. If the individual survives the acute overdose, toxic effects such as sedation and slurred speech may take several weeks to disappear.

Primidone

Primidone (Mysoline) is related to phenobarbital structurally, and it is broken down in part to phenobarbital. Both primidone and its metabolic breakdown products are effective anticonvulsants. Primidone suppresses generalized tonic-clonic (grand mal) and complex partial seizures, but it is not generally the drug of choice for either. It is used for these and other types of seizures if the patient cannot tolerate another drug or if the drug of choice does not provide full seizure control.[5]

Primidone is supplied as a tablet or a syrup and is commonly used in both adults and children. The usual adult dose is 250 milligrams three or four times daily. The dose recommended for children varies with the age and size of the child. Most individuals tolerate this drug best if they start with a small dose once daily and gradually increase the amount they take each day. Sedation limits how quickly the dose can be increased.

Adverse reactions are similar to those with phenobarbital.

People who are allergic to phenobarbital will be allergic to primidone; the allergy may cause little more than a rash, but some patients develop hives (urticaria) or asthma. The therapeutic level of primidone in the serum is 6 to 12 micrograms per milliliter. Toxic and idiosyncratic reactions to this drug include staggering gait, memory disturbances, acute confusion, and delusions of being persecuted. Toxic manifestations may appear much sooner after an oral dose of primidone than after phenobarbital, because peak serum levels of primidone are reached within three hours.

Carbamazepine

Carbamazepine (Tegretol) is the drug of choice for complex partial (psychomotor) seizures and is also effective against simple partial and generalized tonic-clonic seizures. It is available as a tablet. The usual adult dose is one or two 200 milligram tablets three times a day. A serum level of 6 to 10 micrograms per milliliter is usually therapeutic.[6]

Although there was considerable concern when carbamazepine was first introduced that it would cause bleeding disorders, the most frequent toxic reactions are neurological. Dizziness, lightheadedness, and double vision develop as the serum level of the drug increases above the therapeutic range. Some patients experience pins-and-needles sensations and excessive fatigue, which may persist for several days after the drug is stopped. Some patients are allergic to carbamazepine; most have some nausea when they begin taking it. Gastrointestinal discomfort can be minimized by starting at a low dose, such as half a tablet twice a day, and increasing the daily dose until the therapeutic level is reached.

Ethosuximide

Ethosuximide (Zarontin) and related substances, like methsuximide (Celontin), are the drugs of choice in petit mal epilepsy. These drugs are supplied as suspensions or tablets and are usually taken by mouth. The adult dose of ethosuximide is 750 to 2000 milligrams divided into three doses daily. The pediatric dose varies with the size and age of the child. After five or six days of regular use the therapeutic level of 50 to 100 micrograms per milliliter is usually achieved.[7]

Much more common than allergic reactions to this drug are gastrointestinal problems, including nausea, vomiting, and loss of appetite. Toxic and idiosyncratic reactions include acute confusion and mood disturbances. The mood changes may range from apathy and lack of initiative to euphoria. Patients with long-standing intellectual impairment may develop extreme paranoia and aggressiveness. Night terrors may become a substantial problem for children taking this drug. The problems developing with methsuximide are similar to those seen with ethosuximide.

Valproic Acid

Dipropylacetic (valproic) acid (Depakene, Epilim), also marketed as sodium valproate, is unrelated structurally to any other anticonvulsant. It is very effective against several different types of generalized seizure disorders. Except for uncertainty over its side effects, it would be the drug of choice for myoclonic and other types of seizures. It is quite effective against generalized absence and tonic-clonic seizures. In capsules or as a syrup, the usual adult dose is 250 or 500 milligrams four to five times daily.[8]

Toxic effects occurring above the therapeutic range of 50 to 100 micrograms per milliliter include fatigue, nausea, bleeding problems, and liver abnormalities. Much of the initial enthusiasm for this drug has abated as scattered reports have accumulated of liver problems in patients on even low doses. This liver reaction is rare, but when it occurs it can be lethal. Although most patients tolerate valproic acid very well, liver enzymes must be monitored during the first few months of its use. Other side effects include tremors, headache, bedwetting, insomnia, and loss of appetite. These toxic effects clear up rapidly when the drug is stopped.

Benzodiazepines

Benzodiazepines have limited usefulness as anticonvulsants, but there are some notable exceptions. Diazepam (Valium) is extremely effective for short periods when administered intravenously to treat status epilepticus. It is not at all effective as an anticonvulsant when it is taken orally. Clonazepam (Clonopin) is effective against myoclonic seizures. Carbamazepine (Tegretol), already mentioned as a very effective anticonvulsant, is related to this family of drugs. Lorazepam (Ativan) is also used in the treatment of status epilepticus, but its usefulness in other situations is unknown. Chlordiazepoxide (Librium) and oxazepam (Serax) are not used as antiepileptics.

Surgery and Cerebellar Stimulation

Surgical removal of a piece of brain tissue where abnormal electrical activity begins is occasionally effective in controlling epilepsy that cannot be controlled with medication (see Box 11.4). Since any surgery on the brain may produce a new injury that can lead to seizures, removal of brain tissue to control seizures is performed as a last resort. The procedure is feasible only when a distinct piece of brain tissue that is causing the seizures can

---

Box 11.4
Treatment Options

Antiepileptic drugs

Ketogenic diet

Seizure surgery

Cerebellar stimulation

Group therapy

Family group therapy

---

be identified and when removal of the tissue will not cause unacceptable weakness, memory loss, speech difficulty, or other
neurologic deficits. This means that if abnormal electrical activity is limited to an area of the brain that is vital to speech,
the surgery will not be practical. However, surgery has been
very effective for many individuals with intractable seizures and
is a reasonable option when medications have had little or no
impact on the epilepsy.[9]

Some neurosurgeons have attempted to manage seizures arising from several regions of the brain by cutting the corpus callosum, the principal connection between the two sides of the
brain (Figure 11.1). Cutting this bundle of nerve fibers blocks
disruptive signals originating on one side of the brain from
spreading to the other side. This approach is worthwhile for a few
highly selected patients. Whether this type of surgery could be

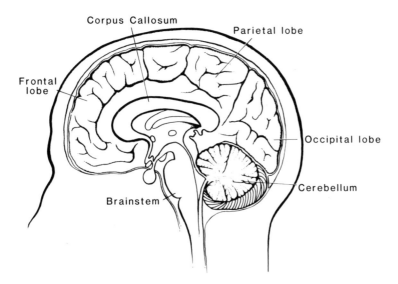

Figure 11.1 Cross-section of the brain. If the right and left sides of
the brain are split apart, a thick band of nerve fibers, the corpus callosum, can be seen. This structure relays information between the
two sides of the brain, but patients can survive after it is cut. The
corpus callosum has been purposely severed in some patients with
intractable seizures, and after the procedure the seizures often abate.

beneficial for a particular patient with intractable seizures is a decision that must involve both the neurosurgeon who will do the procedure and a neurologist who is thoroughly familiar with the patient's disorder.

Seizure surgery, like any other form of neurosurgery, involves substantial risks and is generally appropriate only when the patient can fully understand the risks. Infections, bleeding, and anesthetic mishaps are all possible in even the most competent hands. Some families, exhausted and frustrated after years of recurrent seizure activity, will exert subtle or obvious pressure on the victim of the epilepsy to submit to the surgery. Because no neurologist or neurosurgeon can guarantee that the surgery will control seizures and will not produce new problems, the decision must be strictly the patient's. Conversely, an overprotective family occasionally tries to block the patient's decision to have the surgery. In this situation, too, the patient must be given access to the treatment he or she requests.

The need for thoroughly informed consent presents obvious problems in dealing with a child who might profit from seizure surgery. A 9-year-old who has had poorly controlled seizures for five years is not competent to decide the appropriateness of the neurosurgery. Intellectual development is often significantly impaired by recurrent seizure activity, and the outlook for intellectual improvement is bleak as long as the seizures remain poorly controlled. The child's parents must make an exceedingly difficult decision. If they agree to the surgery, they may feel responsible for an unsatisfactory result, and if they reject the procedure they may suffer considerable guilt as they watch the child continue to have frequent seizures or to deteriorate intellectually. If there are other children in the family, they may be neglected as the parents agonize over whether to subject the epileptic child to surgery. If one parent is less convinced than the other that surgery is essential, the more agreeable parent may be blamed if the surgery produces less than excellent results.

In any decision involving seizure surgery on a child it is essential that the entire family have an opportunity to air questions, fears, and misconceptions. This is not an emergency procedure, and so there is time to allow the parents, and ideally other members of the family as well, to reach a consensus. The fact is that brain surgery in a child with poorly controlled seizures is often very effective, and neurologic deficits appearing after the surgery are often transient. A physician with no vested interest in the procedure, that is, one who will not be involved in the surgery, should discuss the advisability of the procedure with the family. The purpose and character of the surgery should certainly not be concealed from the epileptic child. Efforts to protect the child by keeping him in the dark can lead him to develop terrifying fantasies to explain his ordeal.

Electrical stimulation of the cerebellum, the part of the brain involved primarily in coordination of muscle activity, has been tried in several patients with poorly controlled seizures. This approach has been highly effective in suppressing artificially induced seizure activity in some experimental animals, but the results in people have been less dramatic. The procedure is attractive because little neurosurgery is involved. Enlargement of the opening at the base of the skull is almost all that is needed to allow electrodes to be placed on the surface of the cerebellum. Since most of the output from the cerebellum to the rest of the brain is inhibitory, electrical stimulation of the cerebellum can reasonably be expected to suppress excessive electrical activity in other parts of the brain. This technique is still being evaluated and is undeniably experimental. Unless modifications produce dramatically improved results, it will not be a viable alternative to more conventional seizure surgery.[10]

Diets, Vitamins, and Homeopathic Cures

Everyone faced with a lifelong burden of medication or uncertain seizure control hopes for a simple cure for the seizure disorder. This accounts for the enduring appeal of special diets, vitamin regimens, and other folk remedies that range from voodoo ceremonies to exercise classes. An eyewitness account of a remarkable cure or a dramatic improvement in seizure control is more convincing than bland statistics showing that the effect of the megavitamins, holy water, or self-hypnosis do not exceed what would have been expected on the basis of chance alone. The inexplicable treatment has the allure of magic. After dealing with negative and unexciting doctors, patients find it a relief to hear from proselytizing faddists that little more than an act of faith will cure them.

Logic has no place in efforts to discourage a person with epilepsy from pursuing these unorthodox treatments. The best that anyone can hope for is that the patient will not discontinue an effective treatment in a misguided effort to pursue a simpler remedy.

One diet that does help with seizure control has been recognized for decades. This is the ketogenic diet, one that is high in fats and low in carbohydrates. Raising the level of ketones in the blood by eating a diet consisting mostly of vegetable oils and cream will reduce the seizure threshold in many individuals, but the foods allowed are difficult to tolerate even for a few days and to be effective the diet must be followed for longer periods. The ketogenic diet is usually used as a supplement to anticonvulsant medication for children with minor motor seizures when drugs have failed to suppress seizure activity. It is a dietary approach with documented merit, but the character of the diet guarantees its unacceptability except for the most desperate individuals.[11]

Treatment of Pseudoseizures

Contrived or factitious seizures present special problems for the family. In fact, this is one type of seizure disorder that is much more a problem for people involved with the patient than for the patient himself. The contrived seizure activity is used to gain attention or special consideration, and so it is especially difficult to suppress. Anticonvulsant medication will not affect the frequency and disruptiveness of the attacks until the patient is heavily sedated. Confronting the patient with evidence that the seizure activity is not authentic will not stop the behavior but will undermine the relationship between the physician unmasking the factitious complaint and the patient.

Many people with pseudoseizures have authentic seizures as

well. They may develop the pseudoseizures when they recognize that having a seizure exempts them from a variety of responsibilities and expectations. Reenacting the entire seizure scenario is occasionally helpful in determining what is prompting pseudoseizures. The patient is asked to recreate as much as possible the activity typical of a seizure, and the rest of the family is asked to behave as it customarily does when one occurs. Without the excitement and anxiety of a real episode, the role played by each member of the family becomes more apparent, and what the patient stands to gain by faking a seizure is more easily determined. It may be possible to discourage the pseudoseizures by simple devices, such as requiring that every member of the family, not just the ones who would ordinarily care for the patient, go to the scene when a contrived seizure begins. A child whose nocturnal pseudoseizures have always given her her father's exclusive attention in the middle of the night may find little incentive to have them when the entire family waits by her bed.

In any approach to pseudoseizures a vigilance must be maintained that will not allow the patient to suffer an injury even if the seizure is authentic. With this vigilance must come an even-handed approach to the patient whenever he or she appears sick. The seizure, whether real or contrived, may exempt the patient from responsibilities, such as going to work or to school, but it does not entitle him or her to indulge in leisure activities. After a true seizure a patient may be content to do virtually nothing for several hours, but after a contrived seizure this imposed inactivity may be intolerable. The child who cannot go to school should not be allowed to play games or watch television. It is unwise to make life with seizures entertaining when there is reason to suspect that the seizures are factitious. These seizures should be treated as unfortunate interruptions of the activities planned by the family and not as reasons for canceling plans.

Once steps have been taken to make the drama surrounding the pseudoseizure less rewarding, the patient should be given a reasonable and face-saving way out of the "seizures." A change in medication for a patient who has real seizures as well as contrived ones, suggestions that the problem is resolving itself as a part of its natural course, and information on biofeedback techniques to modify the sensations preceding a pseudoseizure are all strategies available to the patient's physician. The family plays an invaluable role in ending this type of behavior by constantly working to make the behavior unrewarding.

Emergency Management

When a seizure occurs, family members are often obliged to cope with it. If an isolated seizure occurs in a patient who has a well-established seizure disorder, there is usually no need to get emergency medical attention. But if the episode is a change in the individual's usual level of seizure control, the physician should be notified. There is little that anyone—physician, family member, or good samaritan—can do during the seizure to stop it; this is important to remember when people witnessing the seizure run about frantically and insist that something must be done. The principal objective in the management of a seizure is to keep the victim from suffering any injury. If the seizure is a generalized absence (petit mal) episode, the risk of self-injury is negligible. If the seizure is a generalized tonic-clonic (grand mal) seizure or progresses to a generalized convulsion, the risk of injury is much more substantial. Individuals with focal motor or focal sensory seizures may need no assistance during the episode. People with ictal confusion, but no motor problems such as falling to the ground or thrashing limbs, may need little more than careful observation and occasional direction to avoid mishaps.

Avoiding Restraints

Trying to restrain convulsive movements of the limbs or trunk is unnecessary and unwise, since it can injure both the person having the seizure and the person restraining him. A patient with convulsive seizures who realizes that a seizure is about to occur should be helped into a position that will minimize the danger of injury. The best position is usually lying on one's side in a location without nearby objects to fall against or kick. Ideally this means getting the seizure victim onto a padded floor in the middle of an area without furniture. There is little point in having the victim lie on a narrow sofa or sit in a padded chair, since he is likely to fall off. Rather than holding the victim's arms and legs, bystanders should try to clear objects out of his way. With seizures that involve little thrashing about and much strenuous posturing, pillows placed under or around the victim may reduce bruising. If the patient is already unconscious and lying on his back when he is found, it is often a good idea to roll him onto his side to keep him from choking. Changing the patient's position should always be done by pushing or pulling on the trunk, not the limbs, because shoulder dislocations sometimes occur during generalized convulsions.

Limited Use of Tongue Protection

Never force a stick, spoon, or other object into the mouth of a person who is having a seizure. If the jaws are firmly closed, trying to pry them apart with a stiff object may cause more damage than the convulsion itself. Teeth may be dislodged and end up in the lungs, and the tongue or gums may be lacerated. If there is warning that a generalized convulsion is going to occur, a thin but strong and well-padded object, such as a wooden tongue depressor wrapped with gauze, can be placed between the jaws to keep them from closing completely; this may protect the tongue and gums from being bitten. Dentures or other removable dental work should be removed if there is time at the beginning of a seizure.

Avoiding Assisted Breathing

As already mentioned, during generalized convulsions breathing may stop for several seconds or appear very labored, and the patient may turn slightly blue. These changes make witnesses worry that the seizure victim will suffocate. Observers should not attempt to clear the victim's airway. In a minute or two, as the ictus passes, the victim will develop a more normal skin color and breathing pattern. If breathing remains disturbed and the mouth can be opened, obstruction of the airway should be cautiously but rapidly investigated by gently pulling the tongue forward and tilting the head backward. The seizure victim cannot actually "swallow" his tongue, but it may partially obstruct the airway. If the impaired consciousness is from a seizure, resuscitation should not be necessary.

Avoiding Aspiration

Trying to get the seizure victim to drink immediately after the convulsion is pointless and dangerous. The liquid may be inhaled into the lungs, and the cough reflex that would normally limit the damage that such aspirated fluid could cause in the lungs is likely to be defective during the early postictal period. There is no beverage, alcoholic or otherwise, that will speed the victim's recovery from postictal confusion.

Avoiding Premature Activity

Rushing the seizure victim into walking or sitting before the postictal confusion has cleared is also risky. Although seeing the person upright may be reassuring to bystanders, it increases the possibility of a fall. The victim will get up without encouragement when the postictal confusion has passed. If an injury, such as a twisted ankle or a pulled back muscle, has occurred during the seizure, the individual can avoid making it worse much more effectively when he is fully alert than when he is confused.

Recognizing Status Epilepticus

When seizures occur one after another with no return to normal consciousness in between, the individual is said to be in status epilepticus. This is a potentially lethal situation if competent medical treatment is not quickly obtained. In the hands of an experienced neurologist or other physician familiar with its management, status epilepticus is usually completely reversible. Two or three seizures in one day do not constitute status epilepticus, but four or five seizures in one hour are highly suggestive of the problem. Anyone having frequent seizures should be brought to a facility equipped to manage status epilepticus. In most cases, this means a hospital emergency room.

Treatment Changes

Changes in medication on the day that a seizure occurs should always be decided by the patient's physician. Family members often give the patient additional medication immediately after a seizure. The rate at which most antiepileptic drugs are absorbed into the bloodstream is too slow to make this a useful strategy in most cases. Notable exceptions include carbamazepine, primidone, and valproic acid, but the dosages of these medications may already be at maximum beneficial levels when seizures recur, and increasing the number of pills taken may be useless. Because seizures may occur at inopportune times and physicians cannot always be contacted when urgent questions arise, the people who are likely to be present when the patient has a seizure should have a clearly defined plan. What should be done about medication on the day of the seizure, what signs justify a trip to the emergency room, and what questions should be asked after the seizure to help define its cause should all be settled before the seizure occurs, in consultation with the physician.

Group Therapy

People with epilepsy usually profit from the opportunity to meet with similarly affected individuals. Such interactions eliminate the feeling of isolation that often burdens people with a seizure disorder. In group meetings, the deception and fear of discovery that permeate the life of a person with marginally controlled epilepsy can be discarded. Discussing the problems associated with work, family, seizure control, and sexual dysfunction can be very helpful, because people with similar types of epilepsy often have remarkably similar problems.

Self-deprecation is common when patients with epilepsy first enter group discussions, but after a few meetings this abates. These patients feel less impaired when they see what other people with similar problems have done. Alliances between similarly affected patients develop quickly. One young man with complex partial seizures commented, "Meeting other people with the problem gives you the feeling that you are dealing with people understanding the problem" Out of this alliance develop strategies for dealing with the epilepsy.[12]

The belligerence and animosity that often characterize interactions between people with epilepsy and their unaffected peers also abate. As one individual with very poorly controlled epilepsy explained after attending group meetings for several months, "If people can't handle my epilepsy, it's their problem." The patients' resentment that they face special sanctions persists, but their smoldering jealousy of people who do not have epilepsy and the irrepressible self-pity that comes with most chronic disabilities decrease.

When the family of the person with epilepsy is involved in the group, the strains that have developed within the family can be minimized. In a typical family group that met on a regular basis for several months, the most common issues raised included: adjusting to the illness; relieving tension in the family; planning the future; balancing dangers faced willingly by the patient with the desire to feel useful; financial worries; divorce; suicide; changes in social life; living in the present; medication compliance; explaining the illness to other people, including doctors; alternatives to work; and problems with the immediate and extended family.

All of these problems require attention, and solutions to them are not feasible in a strictly medical setting. Finding alternatives to a lifestyle that has had to be abandoned because of the seizure disorder is not the function of a physician or a social worker. The alternatives must come from people who have the problem. Group meetings limited to individuals with epilepsy have the disadvantage of excluding family members, who provide a more objective assessment of what the problems are and how they truly arise. Enabling these families to meet and explore common dilemmas is more likely to minimize the disruptive effects of the seizures than is monitoring serum anticonvulsant levels and adjusting medications. Involving medical personnel in the meeting helps to counteract the erroneous information brought by participating families, and involving a family therapist helps direct the group to real insights. Any family can survive the disruptiveness of poorly controlled epilepsy in one of its members, but no family under this burden should be expected to function productively alone.

Notes

1. Epilepsy: Its Characteristics and Impact

1. W. A. Hauser et al., "Seizure recurrence after a first unprovoked seizure," *New England Journal of Medicine*, 307, no. 9 (1982): 522–528. M. T. Jennings and T. D. Bird, "Genetic influences in the epilepsies," *American Journal of Diseases in Children*, 135 (1981): 450–457.

2. A. T. Reder and F. S. Wright, "Epilepsy evoked by eating: the role of peripheral input," *Neurology* (New York), 32, no. 9 (1982): 1065–1069.

3. G. Burden, "Social aspects," in *Epilepsy and Psychiatry*, ed. E. H. Reynolds and M. R. Trimble (New York: Churchill Livingstone, 1981), pp. 296–305. J. T. Fox, "The epileptic in industry," *British Journal of Physical Medicine*, 11 (1948): 140–144. W. F. Caveness and G. H. Gallup, Jr., "A survey of public attitudes toward epilepsy in 1979 with an indication of trends over the past thirty years," *Epilepsia*, 21 (1980): 509–518.

4. C. G. Long and J. R. Moore, "Parental expectations for their epileptic children," *Journal of Child Psychology and Psychiatry*, 20 (1979): 299–312. W. S. Matthews and G. Barabas, "Suicide and epilepsy: a review of the literature," *Psychosomatics*, 22, no. 6 (1981): 515–524. Caveness and Gallup, "Survey of public attitudes."

5. R. Ryan, K. Kempner, and A. C. Emlen, "The stigma of epilepsy as a self-concept," *Epilepsia*, 21 (1980): 433–444.

6. H. Gastaut, "Clinical and electroencephalographical classification of epileptic seizures," *Epilepsia*, 11 (1970): 102.

7. I. Rapin, *Children with Brain Dysfunction: Neurology, Cognition, Language, and Behavior* (New York: Raven Press, 1982). E. A. Rodin, *The Prognosis of Patients with Epilepsy* (Springfield, Mass.: Charles C.

Thomas, 1968). E. S. Goldensohn and R. Koehle, *EEG Interpretation*, (Mount Kisco, N.Y.: Futura Publishing, 1975). E. S. Goldensohn, "The classification of epileptic seizures," in *The Nervous System*, vol. 2, ed. D. B. Tower (New York: Raven Press, 1975), p. 261.

8. Jennings and Bird, "Genetic influences." Rodin, *Prognosis*.

9. International League against Epilepsy, Commission on Classification and Terminology, "Proposal for the revised clinical and electroencephalographic classification of epileptic seizures," *Epilepsia* 22 (1981): 489–501. Goldensohn, "Classification."

10. D. Blumer, "Temporal lobe epilepsy and its psychiatric significance," in *Psychiatric Aspects of Neurologic Disease*, ed. D. F. Benson and D. Blumer (New York: Grune and Stratton, 1975), p. 171.

11. S. G. Waxman and N. Geschwind, "The interictal behavior syndrome of temporal lobe epilepsy," *Archives of General Psychiatry*, 32 (1975): 1580–1586. Goldensohn, "Classification." A. V. Delgado-Escueta, D. M. Treiman, and G. O. Walsh, "The treatable epilepsies (part 2)," *New England Journal of Medicine*, 308, no. 26 (1983): 1576–1584.

12. A. Hecker, F. Andermann, and E. A. Rodin, "Spitting automatism in temporal lobe seizures," *Epilepsia*, 13 (1972): 767–772. E. S. Goldensohn and A. P. Gold, "Prolonged behavioral disturbances as ictal phenomena," *Neurology*, 10 (1959): 767. P. Flor-Henry, "Ictal and interictal psychiatric manifestations in epilepsy: specific or non-specific?" *Epilepsia*, 13 (1972): 773–783. Delgado-Escueta, Treiman, and Walsh, "Treatable epilepsies."

13. Hecker, Andermann, and Rodin, "Spitting automatism." R. R. Babb and P. B. Eckman, "Abdominal epilepsy," *Journal of the American Medical Association*, 222 (1972): 65–66. G. M. Remillard et al., "Water-drinking as ictal behavior in complex partial seizures," *Neurology*, 31 (1981): 117–124.

14. E. Slater and A. W. Beard, "The schizophrenia-like psychoses of epilepsy. 1. Psychiatric aspects," *British Journal of Psychiatry*, 109 (1963): 95–150. Flor-Henry, "Ictal and interictal psychiatric manifestations." K. J. Mohan, M. W. Salo, and S. Nagaswami, "A case of limbic system dysfunction with hypersexuality and fugue state," *Diseases of the Nervous System*, 36 (1975): 621–624. R. S. McLachlan and W. T. Blume, "Isolated fear in complex partial status epilepticus," *Annals of Neurology*, 8 (1980): 639–641.

15. Blumer, "Temporal lobe epilepsy."

16. E. A. Rodin, "Psychosocial management of patients with complex partial seizures," in *Advances in Neurology*, vol. 11, ed. J. K. Penry and D. D. Daly (New York: Raven Press, 1975), p. 383. Slater and Beard,

"Schizophrenia-like psychoses." Blumer, "Temporal lobe epilepsy." Remillard, Andermann, and Gloor, "Water-drinking," p. 117.

17. N. Malamud, "Psychiatric disorder with intracranial tumors of the limbic system," *Archives of Neurology*, 17 (1967): 113–123. Goldensohn and Gold, "Prolonged behavioral disturbances." Mohan, Salo, and Nagaswami, "Limbic system dysfunction," p. 621. Blumer, "Temporal lobe epilepsy." J. Gunn, "Violence and epilepsy," *New England Journal of Medicine*, 306 (1982): 298–299.

18. Blumer, "Temporal lobe epilepsy."

19. H. E. Booker, "Management of the difficult patient with complex partial seizures," in *Advances in Neurology*, vol. 11, ed. Penry and Daly, p. 369. S. G. Waxman and N. Geschwind, "Hypergraphia in temporal lobe epilepsy," *Neurology*, 24 (1974): 629–636. Flor-Henry, "Ictal and interictal psychiatric manifestations," p. 773.

20. League against Epilepsy, "Proposal for Revised Classification." Goldensohn and Koehle, *EEG Interpretation*. Goldensohn, "Classification."

21. Rapin, *Children with Brain Dysfunction.*

2. The Adult with Epilepsy

1. T. Okuma and H. Kumashiro, "Natural history and prognosis of epilepsy: report of a multi-institutional study in Japan," *Epilepsia*, 22 (1981): 35–53.

2. Ibid.

3. M. Mailick, "The impact of severe illness on the individual and family: an overview," *Social Work and Health Care*, 5, no. 2 (1979): 117–128. R. G. Feldman and N. L. Paul, "Identity of emotional triggers in epilepsy," *Journal of Nervous and Mental Diseases*, 162, no. 5 (1976): 345–353.

4. Information in this section from the following sources: B. Bursten and R. D'Esopo, "The obligation to remain sick," *Archives of General Psychiatry*, 12, no. 4 (1965): 402–407. B. Bursten, "Family dynamics, the sick role, and medical hospital admissions," *Family Process*, 4, no. 2 (1965): 206–216. Mailick, "Impact of severe illness." N. F. Bracht, "The social nature of chronic disease and disability," *Social Work and Health Care*, 5, no. 2 (1979): 129–144.

5. Information in this section from the following sources: S. E. Lessman and L. R. Mollick, "Group treatment of epileptics," *Health and Social Work*, 3, no. 3 (1978): 106–121. R. A. Pigott, *Evaluation of a Service Program Focused on Vocational Rehabilitation as Prototype for*

an Urban Voluntary Epilepsy Agency (Boston: Epilepsy Society of Massachusetts, 1969). R. P. Schwartz, "Epilepsy employment: a historical perspective," in *The Commission for the Control of Epilepsy and Its Consequences: Plan for Nationwide Action on Epilepsy*, vol. 2 (Washington, D.C.: Department of Health, Education, and Welfare, 1977), pp. 491–546.

6. Information in this section from the following sources: Schwartz, "Epilepsy employment." E. A. Rodin, *The Prognosis of Patients with Epilepsy* (Springfield, Mass.: Charles C. Thomas, 1968). Pigott, *Evaluation of a Service Program*. Bracht, "Chronic disease." W. F. Caveness and G. H. Gallup, Jr., "A survey of public attitudes toward epilepsy in 1979 with an indication of trends over the past thirty years," *Epilepsia*, 21 (1980): 509–518.

7. B. K. Jerath and B. A. Kimbell, "Hospitalization rates for epilepsy in the United States, 1973–1976," *Epilepsia*, 22 (1981): 55–64. Bursten, "Family dynamics."

8. C. B. Dodrill et al., "An objective method for the assessment of psychological and social problems among epileptics," *Epilepsia*, 21 (1980): 123–135.

9. Schwartz, "Epilepsy employment."

10. Rodin, *Prognosis*. B. O. Berg, "Prognosis of childhood epilepsy—another look," *New England Journal of Medicine*, 306, no. 14 (1982): 861–862.

11. Information in this section from the following sources: W. A. Hauser, J. F. Annegers, and L. R. Elveback, "Mortality in patients with epilepsy," *Epilepsia*, 21 (1980): 399–412. L. A. Woodbury, "Shortening of the lifespan and mortality of patients with epilepsy," in *Plan for Nationwide Action on Epilepsy*, vol. 4 (Washington, D.C.: Commission for the Control of Epilepsy and Its Consequences, 1978). B. Barraclough, "Suicide and epilepsy," in *Epilepsy and Psychiatry*, ed. E. H. Reynolds and M. R. Trimble (New York: Churchill Livingstone, 1981), pp. 72–76. J. J. Zielinski, "Epilepsy and mortality rate and cause of death," *Epilepsia*, 16 (1974): 191–201.

3. Marital Problems

1. T. Tsuboi, "Incidence of seizures among offspring of epileptic patients," in *Epilepsy, Pregnancy, and the Child*, ed. D. Janz et al. (New York: Raven Press, 1982), pp. 527–534.

2. L. V. Dansky, E. Andermann, and F. Andermann, "Marriage and fertility in epileptic patients," *Epilepsia*, 21 (1980): 261–271. J. Lindsay,

C. Ounsted, and P. Richards, "Long-term outcome in children with temporal lobe seizures. II. Marriage, parenthood and sexual indifference," *Developmental Medicine and Child Neurology*, 21 (1979): 433–440.

4. Sexual Activity

1. D. Blumer, "Temporal lobe epilepsy and its psychiatric significance," in *Psychiatric Aspects of Neurologic Disease*, ed. D. F. Benson and D. Blumer (New York, Grune and Stratton, 1975), p. 171.

2. D. C. Taylor, "Sexual behavior and temporal lobe epilepsy," *Archives of Neurology*, 21 (1969): 510–516. J. Lindsay, C. Ounsted, and P. Richards, "Long-term outcome in children with temporal lobe seizures. II. Marriage, parenthood and sexual indifference," *Developmental Medicine and Child Neurology*, 21 (1979): 433–440. S. G. Waxman and N. Geschwind, "The interictal behavior syndrome of temporal lobe epilepsy," *Archives of General Psychiatry*, 32 (1975): 1580–1586. Blumer, "Temporal lobe epilepsy."

3. Waxman and Geschwind, "Interictal behavior." R. Hunter, V. Logue, and W. H. McMenimy, "Temporal lobe epilepsy supervening on long-standing transvestism and fetishism," *Epilepsia*, 4 (1973): 60–65. A. Kolarsky et al., "Male sexual deviation: association with early temporal lobe damage," *Archives of General Psychiatry*, 17 (1976): 735–743. G. M. Remillard et al., "Sexual ictal manifestations predominate in women with temporal lobe epilepsy: a finding suggesting sexual dimorphism in the human brain," *Neurology* (Cleveland), 33, no. 3 (1983): 323–330. R. D. Currier, et al., "Sexual seizures," *Archives of Neurology*, 25 (1971): 260–264.

4. Information in this section from the following sources: Remillard ed al., "Sexual ictal manifestations." Kolarsky et al., "Male sexual deviation."

5. Childbearing and Inheritance

1. Information in this section from the following sources: L. V. Dansky, E. Andermann, and F. Andermann, "Marriage and fertility in epileptic patients," *Epilepsia*, 21 (1980): 261–271. J. Lindsay, C. Ounsted, and P. Richards, "Long-term outcome in children with temporal lobe seizures. II. Marriage, parenthood and sexual indifference," *Developmental Medicine and Child Neurology*, 21 (1979): 433–440.

2. Information in this section from the following sources: Y. Nakane et al., "Multi-institutional study on the teratogenicity and fetal

toxicity of antiepileptic drugs: a report of a collaborative study group in Japan," *Epilepsia*, 21 (1980): 663–680. M. C. Phelan, J. M. Pellock, and E. W. Nance, "Discordant expression of fetal hydantoin syndrome in heteropaternal dizygotic twins," *New England Journal of Medicine*, 307 (1982): 99–101.

3. Information in this section from the following sources: M. T. Jennings and T. D. Bird, "Genetic influences in the epilepsies," *American Journal of Diseases of Children*, 135 (1981): 450–457. D. Janz et al., "Epilepsy in children of epileptic parents," in *Epilepsy, Pregnancy, and the Child*, ed. D. Janz et al. (New York: Raven Press, 1982), pp. 527–534. T. Tsuboi, "Incidence of seizures among offspring of epileptic patients," in *Epilepsy, Pregnancy, and the Child*, ed Janz et al., pp. 503–507. D. Blumer, "Temporal lobe epilepsy and its psychiatric significance," in *Psychiatric Aspects of Neurologic Disease*, ed. D. F. Benson and D. Blumer (New York: Grune and Stratton, 1975), p. 171.

4. Information in this section from the following sources: I. Rapin, *Children with Brain Dysfunction: Neurology, Cognition, Language, and Behavior* (New York: Raven Press, 1982). Jennings and Bird, "Genetic influences." K. B. Nelson and J. H. Ellenberg, "Predictors of epilepsy in children who have experienced febrile seizures," *New England Journal of Medicine*, 295, no. 19 (1976): 1029–1033. T. W. Farmer and R. S. Greenwood, "Paroxysmal disorders," in *Pediatric Neurology*, ed. T. W. Farmer (Philadelphia: Harper and Row, 1983), pp. 205–263.

5. Information in this section from the following sources: Jennings and Bird, "Genetic influences." C. F. Barlow, *Mental Retardation and Related Disorders* (Philadelphia: F. A. Davis, 1978). J. J. Volpe, *Neurology of the Newborn* (Philadelphia: W. B. Saunders, 1981), pp. 357–403. J. E. Etheridge, Jr., "Birth defects and developmental disorders," in *Pediatric Neurology*, ed. Farmer, pp. 61–115. J. U. Toglia, M. Mc-Glamery, and R. R. Sambandham, "Tetrabenazine in the treatment of Huntington's chorea and other hyperkinetic movement disorders," *Journal of Clinical Psychiatry*, 39 (1978): 81–87.

6. Children with Epilepsy

1. B. O. Berg, "Prognosis of childhood epilepsy—another look," *New England Journal of Medicine*, 306, no. 14 (1982): 861–862. C. Appolone, "Preventive social work intervention with families of children with epilepsy," *Social Work and Health Care*, 4, no. 2 (1978): 139–148. R. G. Ziegler, "Impairments of control and competence in epileptic children and their families," *Epilepsia*, 22 (1981): 339–346. G. Burden, "Social aspects," in *Epilepsy and Psychiatry*, ed. E. H. Reynolds and

M. R. Trimble (New York: Churchill Livingstone, 1981), pp. 296–305.

2. Ziegler, "Impairments." K. Ritchie, "Research note: interaction in the families of epileptic children," *Journal of Child Psychology and Psychiatry*, 22 (1981): 65–71.

3. D. Pond, "Psycho-social aspects of epilepsy—the family," in *Epilepsy and Psychiatry*, ed. Reynolds and Trimble, pp. 291–295.

4. W. A. Hauser et al., "Seizure recurrence after a first unprovoked seizure," *New England Journal of Medicine*, 307, no. 9 (1982): 522–528.

5. M. T. Jennings and T. D. Bird, "Genetic influences in the epilepsies," *American Journal of Diseases of Children*, 135 (1981): 450–457.

6. E. A. Rodin, *The Prognosis of Patients with Epilepsy* (Springfield, Mass.: Charles C. Thomas, 1968). F. A. Gutierrez and A. J. Raimondi, "Acute subdural hematoma in infancy and childhood," *Child's Brain*, 1 (1975): 269–290.

7. Information in this section from the following sources: Berg, "Prognosis." "Febrile convulsions," *British Medical Journal*, 282, no. 6265 (1981): 673–674. K. B. Nelson and J. H. Ellenberg, "Predictors of epilepsy in children who have experienced febrile seizures," *New England Journal of Medicine*, 295, no. 19 (1976): 1029–1033. J. H. Thurston et al., "Prognosis in childhood epilepsy," *New England Journal of Medicine*, 307, no. 9 (1982): 555. Jennings and Bird, "Genetic influences." F. A. Bassen and A. L. Kornzweig, "Malformation of the erythrocytes in a case of atypical retinitis pigmentosa, *Blood*, 5 (1950): 381–387.

8. K. R. Mahaffey et al., "National estimates of blood levels: United States, 1976–1980," *New England Journal of Medicine*, 307, no. 10 (1982): 573–579. J. S. Lin-Fu, "Children and lead: new findings and concerns," *New England Journal of Medicine*, 307, no. 10 (1982): 615–616.

9. S. Gilman, J. Bloedel, R. Lechtenberg, *Disorders of the Cerebellum* (Philadelphia: F. A. Davis, 1981).

10. R. Lechtenberg, *The Psychiatrist's Guide to Diseases of the Nervous System* (New York: John Wiley, 1982).

11. Information in this section from the following sources: B. P. Hermann, R. B. Black, and S. Chabria, "Behavioral problems and social competence in children with epilepsy," *Epilepsia*, 22 (1981): 703–710. C. G. Long and J. R. Moore, "Parental expectations for their epileptic children," *Journal of Child Psychology and Psychiatry* 20 (1979): 299–312. Appolone, "Preventive social work."

12. Hermann, Black, and Chabria, "Behavioral problems." B. P. Hermann et al., "Aggression and epilepsy: seizure-type comparisons and high-risk variables," *Epilepsia*, 21 (1980): 692–698. Appolone, "Preventive social work."

13. Information in this section from the following sources: Appo-

lone, "Preventive social work." D. S. O'Leary et al., "Effects of age of onset of tonic-clonic seizures on neuropsychological performance in children," *Epilepsia*, 22 (1981): 197–204. Burden, "Social aspects." C. F. Barlow, *Mental Retardation and Related Disorders* (Philadelphia: F. A. Davis, 1978). Long and Moore, "Parental expectations."

14. Information in this section from the following sources: S. E. Lessman and L. R. Mollick, "Group treatment of epileptics," *Health and Social Work*, 3, no. 3 (1978): 106–121. Appolone, "Preventive social work." Long and Moore, "Parental expectations."

15. Information in this section from the following sources: "Drugs for epilepsy," *Medical Letter on Drugs and Therapeutics*, 25, no. 643 (1983): 81–84. G. Tollefson, "Psychiatric implications of anticonvulsant drugs," *Journal of Clinical Psychiatry*, 41 (1980): 295. H. E. Booker, "Management of the difficult patient with complex partial seizures," in *Advances in Neurology*, vol. 11, ed. J. K. Penry and D. D. Daly (New York: Raven Press, 1975), p. 369. J. K. Penry and M. E. Newmark, "The use of antiepileptic drugs," *Annals of Internal Medicine*, 90 (1979): 207. R. D. Franks and A. J. Richter, "Schizophrenia-like psychosis associated with anticonvulsant toxicity," *American Journal of Psychiatry*, 136 (1979): 973. Rodin, *Prognosis*.

16. Information in this section from the following sources: Ziegler, "Impairments." T. P. Berney et al., "Effects of discotheque environment on epileptic children," *British Medical Journal*, 282, no. 6259 (1981): 180–182. Long and Moore, "Parental expectations." M. E. Lamb, "Paternal influences on early socio-emotional development," *Journal of Child Psychology and Psychiatry*, 23 (1982): 185–190. Ritchie, "Research note."

17. Information in this section from the following sources: Appolone, "Preventive social work." Ziegler, "Impairments."

18. Information in this section from the following sources: Ziegler, "Impairments." Long and Moore, "Parental expectations." Appolone, "Preventive social work." Berney et al., "Discotheque environment." Pond, "Psycho-social aspects." Ritchie, "Research note."

19. Appolone, "Preventive social work." Ziegler, "Impairments." Pond, "Psycho-social aspects."

20. Rodin, *Prognosis*.

21. Information in this section from the following sources: Hauser et al., "Seizure recurrence." B. Jennett, "Epilepsy after head injury and craniotomy," in *Driving and epilepsy*, ed. R. B. Godwin-Austen and M. L. E. Espir, Royal Society of Medicine International Congress and Symposium Series, no. 60 (London: Academic Press, 1983), pp. 49–51.

Rodin, *Prognosis.* Burden, "Social aspects." J. H. Thurston et al., "Prognosis in childhood epilepsy," *New England Journal of Medicine*, 306, no. 14 (1982): 831–836.

22. W. A. Hauser, J. F. Annegers, and L. R. Elveback, "Mortality in patients with epilepsy," *Epilepsia*, 21 (1980): 399–412. B. Barraclough, "Suicide and epilepsy," in *Epilepsy and Psychiatry*, ed. E. H. Reynolds and M. R. Trimble (New York: Churchill Livingstone, 1981), pp. 72–76.

7. Children Growing Up with an Epileptic Parent

1. M. E. Lamb, "Paternal influences on early socio-emotional development," *Journal of Child Psychology and Psychiatry*, 23 (1982): 185–190. W. F. Caveness and G. H. Gallup, Jr., "A survey of public attitudes toward epilepsy in 1979 with an indication of trends over the past thirty years," *Epilepsia*, 21 (1980): 509–518.
2. Lamb, "Paternal influences."
3. Caveness and Gallup, "Survey."

8. Siblings and the Extended Family

1. K. Ritchie, "Research note: interaction in the families of epileptic children," *Journal of Child Psychology and Psychiatry*, 22 (1981): 65–71.

9. Personality Changes and Violence

1. J. Gunn, "Violence and epilepsy," *New England Journal of Medicine*, 306 (1982): 298–299.
2. C. B. Dodrill et al., "An objective method for the assessment of psychological and social problems among epileptics," *Epilepsia*, 21 (1980): 123–135.
3. Ibid. R. Ryan, K. Kempner, and A. C. Emlen, "The stigma of epilepsy as a self-concept," *Epilepsia*, 21 (1980): 433–444.
4. B. P. Hermann et al., "Psychopathology in epilepsy: relationship of seizure type to age at onset," *Epilepsia*, 21 (1980): 15–23.
5. D. M. Bear and P. Fedio, "Quantitative analysis of interictal behavior in temporal lobe epilepsy," *Archives of Neurology*, 32 (1977): 454–467. D. Blumer, "Temporal lobe epilepsy and its psychiatric significance," in *Psychiatric Aspects of Neurologic Disease*, ed. D. F. Benson and D. Blumer (New York: Grune and Stratton, 1975), p. 171. K. Haw-

ton, J. Fagg, and P. Marsack, "Association between epilepsy and attempted suicide," *Journal of Neurology, Neurosurgery and Psychiatry*, 43 (1980): 168–170. E. Slater and A. W. Beard, "The schizophrenia-like psychoses of epilepsy: psychiatric aspects," *British Journal of Psychiatry*, 109 (1963): 95–150. E. A. Serafetinides, "Aggressiveness in temporal lobe epileptics and its relation to cerebral dysfunction and environmental factors," *Epilepsia*, 6 (1965): 33–42. Bear and Fedio, "Quantitative analysis."

6. Slater and Beard, "Psychoses." E. Valenstein and K. M. Heilman, "Emotional disorders resulting from lesions of the central nervous system," in *Clinical Neuropsychology*, ed. K. M. Heilman and E. Valenstein (New York: Oxford University Press, 1979), p. 413.

7. Blumer, "Temporal lobe epilepsy." N. F. Bracht, "The social nature of chronic disease and disability," *Social Work and Health Care*, 5, no. 2 (1979): 129–144.

8. E. Strauss, A. Risser, and M. W. Jones, "Fear responses in patients with epilepsy," *Archives of Neurology*, 39, no. 10 (1982): 626–630.

9. K. Poeck, "Pathophysiology of emotional disorders associated with brain damage," in *Handbook of Clinical Neurology*, vol. 3, ed. P. J. Vinken and G. W. Bruyn (New York: American Elsevier, 1969), p. 343. M. Goldstein, "Brain research and violent behavior," *Archives of Neurology*, 30 (1974): 1–34.

10. J. H. Pincus, "Can violence be a manifestation of epilepsy?" *Neurology*, 30 (1980): 304. Blumer, "Temporal lobe epilepsy." Gunn, "Violence."

11. B. P. Hermann et al., "Aggression and epilepsy: seizure-type comparisons and high-risk variables," *Epilepsia*, 21 (1980): 691–698. J. R. Stevens, "Interictal clinical manifestations of complex partial seizures," in *Advances in Neurology*, vol. 11, ed. J. K. Penry and D. D. Daly (New York: Raven Press, 1975), p. 85.

12. M. A. Falconer, "Reversibility by temporal-lobe resection of the behavioral abnormalities of temporal-lobe epilepsy," *New England Journal of Medicine*, 289 (1973): 451. Hermann et al., "Aggression." Stevens, "Complex partial seizures."

13. Stevens, "Complex partial seizures." D. C. Taylor, "Aggression and epilepsy," *Journal of Psychosomatic Research*, 13 (1969): 229. B. P. Hermann, R. B. Black, and S. Chabria, "Behavioral problems and social competence in children with epilepsy," *Epilepsia*, 22 (1981): 703–710. Hermann et al., "Aggression."

14. R. Mayeux et al., "Interictal memory and language impairment in temporal lobe epilepsy," *Neurology*, 30 (1980): 120.

15. Blumer, "Temporal lobe epilepsy." E. A. Rodin, "Psychosocial management of patients with complex partial seizures," in *Advances in Neurology*, vol. 11, ed. Penry and Daly, p. 383.

16. Hermann et al., "Aggression."

17. Information in this section from the following sources: Gunn, "Violence." B. M. Maletzky, "The episodic dyscontrol syndrome," *Diseases of the Nervous System*, 34 (1973): 178–185. G. Bach-Y-Rita et al., "Episodic dyscontrol: a study of 130 violent patients," *American Journal of Psychiatry*, 127 (1971): 1473. Pincus, "Violence." Goldstein, "Brain research."

18. Blumer, "Temporal lobe epilepsy."

19. Information in this section from the following sources: Hawton, Fagg, and Marsack, "Epilepsy and attempted suicide," pp. 168–170. B. Barraclough, "Suicide and epilepsy," in *Epilepsy and Psychiatry*, ed. E. H. Reynolds and M. R. Trimble (New York: Churchill Livingstone, 1981), pp. 72–76. L. A. Woodbury, "Shortening of the lifespan and mortality of patients with epilepsy," in *Plan for Nationwide Action on Epilepsy*, vol. 4 (Washington, D.C.: Commission for the Control of Epilepsy and Its Consequences, 1978). J. J. Zielinski, "Epilepsy and mortality rate and cause of death," *Epilepsia* 16 (1974): 191–201. W. A. Hauser, J. F. Annegers, and L. R. Elveback, "Mortality in patients with epilepsy," *Epilepsia*, 21 (1980): 399–412. W. S. Matthews and G. Barabas, "Suicide and epilepsy: a review of the literature," *Psychosomatics*, 22, no. 6 (1981): 515–524. A. Mackay, "Self-poisoning—a complication of epilepsy," *British Journal of Psychiatry*, 134 (1979): 277–282.

10. Investigating the Person with Epilepsy

1. W. A. Hauser et al., "Seizure recurrence after a first unprovoked seizure," *New England Journal of Medicine*, 307, no. 9 (1982): 522–528.

2. H. E. Booker, "Management of the difficult patient with complex partial seizures," in *Advances in Neurology*, vol. 11, ed. J. K. Penry and D. D. Daly (New York: Raven press, 1975), p. 63.

3. R. N. Harner, "EEG evaluation of the patient with dementia," in *Psychiatric Aspects of Neurologic Disease*, ed. D. F. Benson and D. Blumer (New York: Grune and Stratton, 1975), p. 63.

4. Ibid. American Psychiatric Association, Task Force on Nomenclature and Statistics, *Diagnostic and Statistical Manual of Mental Disorders*, 3rd ed. (Washington, D.C.: American Psychiatric Association, 1980). R. A. DeVaul and R. C. W. Hall, "Hallucinations," in *Psychiatric Presentations of Medical Illness*, ed. R. C. W. Hall (New York: SP Medical

and Scientific Books, 1980), p. 91. E. S. Goldensohn and R. Koehle, *EEG Interpretation* (Mount Kisco, N.Y.: Futura Publishing, 1975).

5. Hauser et al., "Seizure recurrence."

6. B. Anziska and R. Q. Cracco, "Short latency somatosensory evoked potentials: studies in patients with focal neurological disease," *Electroencephalography and Clinical Neurophysiology*, 49 (1980): 227–239.

7. Hauser et al., "Seizure recurrence." Booker, "Management of the difficult patient."

8. G. Karpati and B. Frame, "Neuropsychiatric disorders in primary hyperparathyroidism," *Archives of Neurology*, 10 (1964): 387. Hauser et al., "Seizure recurrence."

9. Hauser et al., "Seizure recurrence."

10. Ibid.

11. J. A. N. Corsellis, G. J. Goldberg, and A. R. Norton, " 'Limbic encephalitis' and its association with carcinoma," *Brain*, 91 (1968): 481–496.

12. R. Lechtenberg and G. A. Vaida, "Schistosomiasis of the spinal cord," *Neurology* (Minneapolis), 27 (1977): 55–59.

13. R. Bennett et al., "Neuropsychiatric problems in systemic lupus erythematosus," *British Medical Journal*, 4 (1972): 342.

14. Karpati and Frame, "Neuropsychiatric disorders," p. 387. Hauser et al., "Seizure recurrence."

15. Information in this section from M. E. Hillbom, "Occurrence of cerebral seizures provoked by alcohol abuse," *Epilepsia*, 21 (1980): 459–466.

16. Information in this section from the following sources: E. W. Massey and T. L. Riley, "Pseudoseizures: recognition and treatment," *Psychosomatics* 21 (1980): 987. D. W. King et al., "Pseudoseizures: diagnostic evaluation," *Neurology*, 32 (1982): 18–23. A. Roy, "Hysterical seizures," *Archives of Neurology*, 36 (1979): 447. T. A. Gulick, I. P. Spinks, and D. W. King, "Pseudoseizures: ictal phenomena," *Neurology* (New York), 32 (1982): 24–30. M. T. Jennings and T. D. Bird, "Genetic influences in the epilepsies," *American Journal of Diseases of Children*, 135 (1981): 450–457.

11. Treatment

1. Information in this section from the following sources: A. V. Delgado-Escueta, D. M. Treiman and G. O. Walsh, "The treatable epilepsies (second of two parts)," *New England Journal of Medicine*, 308, no. 26 (1983): 1576–1584. T. Okuma and H. Kumashiro, "Natural history and prognosis of epilepsy: report of a multi-institutional study in

Japan," *Epilepsia*, 22 (1981): 35–53. E. A. Rodin, *The Prognosis of Patients with Epilepsy* (Springfield, Mass.: Charles C. Thomas, 1968). B. Jennett, "Epilepsy after head injury and craniotomy," in *Driving and Epilepsy*, ed. R. B. Godwin-Austen and M. L. E. Espir, Royal Society of Medicine International Congress and Symposium Series, no. 60 (London: Academic Press, 1983), pp. 49–51.

2. Information in this section from the following sources: Rodin, *Prognosis*. Delgado-Escueta, Treiman, and Walsh, "Treatable epilepsies."

3. Information on phenytoin from the following sources: "Drugs for epilepsy," *Medical Letter on Drugs and Therapeutics*, 25, no. 643 (1983): 81–84. Delgado-Escueta, Treiman, and Walsh, "Treatable epilepsies." L. W. McLain, J. T. Martin, and J. H. Allen, "Cerebellar degeneration due to chronic phenytoin therapy," *Annals of Neurology*, 7 (1980): 18–23. J. K. Penry and M. E. Newmark, "The use of antiepileptic drugs," *Annals of Internal Medicine*, 90 (1979): 207–218. H. E. Booker, "Management of the difficult patient with complex partial seizures," in *Advances in Neurology*, vol. 11, ed. J. K. Penry and D. D. Daly (New York: Raven Press, 1975), p. 369. R. D. Franks and A. J. Richter, "Schizophrenia-like psychosis associated with anticonvulsant toxicity," *American Journal of Psychiatry*, 136 (1979): 973. R. Lechtenberg, *The Psychiatrist's Guide to Diseases of the Nervous System* (New York: John Wiley, 1982). G. Tollefson, "Psychiatric implications of anticonvulsant drugs," *Journal of Clinical Psychiatry*, 41 (1980): 295–302.

4. Information on phenobarbital from the following sources: "Drugs for epilepsy." Delgado-Escueta, Treiman, and Walsh, "Treatable epilepsies." Tollefson, "Anticonvulsant drugs." Penry and Newmark, "Antiepileptic drugs." Booker, "Complex partial seizures."

5. Information on primidone from the following sources: Penry and Newmark, "Antiepileptic drugs." Tollefson, "Anticonvulsant drugs." Booker, "Complex partial seizures."

6. Information on carbamazepine from the following sources: Booker, "Complex partial seizures." Penry and Newmark, "Antiepileptic drugs." "Drugs for epilepsy." Tollefson, "Anticonvulsant drugs."

7. Information on ethosuximide from the following sources: Booker, "Complex partial seizures." Tollefson, "Anticonvulsant drugs." "Drugs for epilepsy."

8. Information on valproic acid from the following sources: "Drugs for epilepsy." J. Bruni and B. J. Wilder, "Valproic acid," *Archives of Neurology*, 36 (1979): 393–398. Delgado-Escueta, Treiman, and Walsh, "Treatable epilepsies."

9. Delgado-Escueta, Treiman, and Walsh, "Treatable epilepsies."

D. L. Schomer, "Partial epilepsy," *New England Journal of Medicine,* 309, no. 9 (1983): 536–539.

10. M. Riklan, C. Kabat, and I. S. Cooper, "Psychological effects of short term cerebellar stimulation in epilepsy," *Journal of Nervous and Mental Diseases,* 162, no. 4 (1976): 282–290.

11. S. Gilman, J. R. Bloedel, and R. Lechtenberg, *Disorders of the Cerebellum* (Philadelphia: F. A. Davis, 1981). J. Engel, Jr., et al., "Recent developments in the diagnosis and therapy of epilepsy," *Annals of Internal Medicine,* 97 (1982): 584–598.

12. S. E. Lessman and L. R. Mollick, "Group treatment of epileptics," *Health and Social Work,* 3, no. 3 (1978): 106–121.

Index